TRIATHLON
FOR MASTERS
AND BEYOND

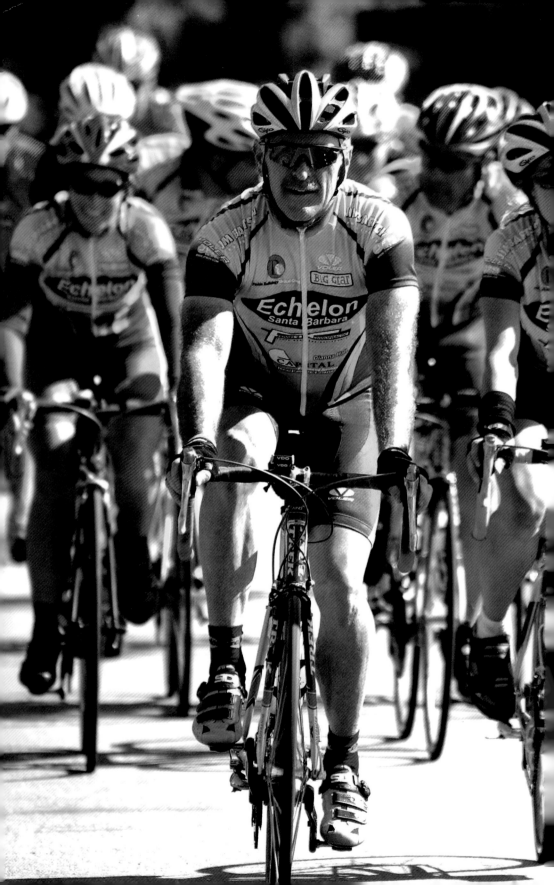

IAN STOKELL

TRIATHLON
FOR MASTERS
AND BEYOND

BLOOMSBURY
LONDON • NEW DELHI • NEW YORK • SYDNEY

Note

While every effort has been made to ensure that the content of this book is as technically accurate and as sound as possible, neither the author nor the publishers can accept responsibility for any injury or loss sustained as a result of the use of this material.

Published by Bloomsbury Publishing Plc
50 Bedford Square
London WC1B 3DP
www.bloomsbury.com

First edition 2013

Copyright © 2013 Ian Stokell

ISBN (print): 978 1 4081 8719 7
ISBN (Epub): 978 1 4729 0246 7
ISBN (Epdf): 978 1 4729 0247 4

A CIP catalogue record for this book is available from the British Library.

Acknowledgements
Cover photographs © Getty Images
Inside photographs: pp. vi, 7, 8, 16, 22, 26, 34, 50, 55, 81, 107, 136, 144, 149, 152, 160, 164–5, 172 and 180 © Getty Images; pp. 2, 13, 53, 58, 62, 66, 70, 83, 92, 120–1, 157 and 177 © Shutterstock; p. ii © Byron W. Moore/Shutterstock.com; pp. viii, 5, 45 and 142–3 © Rihardzz/Shutterstock.com; pp. 31, 86 and 93–4, 110 and 128 © Maxisport/Shutterstock.com; p. 36 © irabel8/Shutterstock.com; pp. 46 and 128 © GTS Production/Shutterstock.com; p. 74 © Stefan Holm/Shutterstock.com; p.76 © ARZTSAMUI/Shutterstock.com; p. 102 © ema/Shutterstock.com; p. 104 © Nicholas Piccillo/Shutterstock.com; pp. 113–4 © Alan C. Heison/Shutterstock.com; p. 118 © Lemonpink images/Shutterstock.com; pp. 124–5 © Martin Good/Shutterstock.com; p. 134 © Daniel Wiedermann/Shutterstock.com; p. 139 © J. Henning Buchholz/Shutterstock.com; p. 155 © Richard Thornton/Shutterstock.com; pp. 168–9 © catwalker/Shutterstock.com
Commissioning Editor: Charlotte Croft
Editor: Sarah Cole
Illustrator: David Gardner

This book is produced using paper that is made from wood grown in managed, sustainable forests. It is natural, renewable and recyclable. The logging and manufacturing processes conform to the environmental regulations of the country of origin.

Typeset in URW Grotesk by seagulls.net

Printed and bound in China by C&C Offset Printing Co

10 9 8 7 6 5 4 3 2 1

CONTENTS

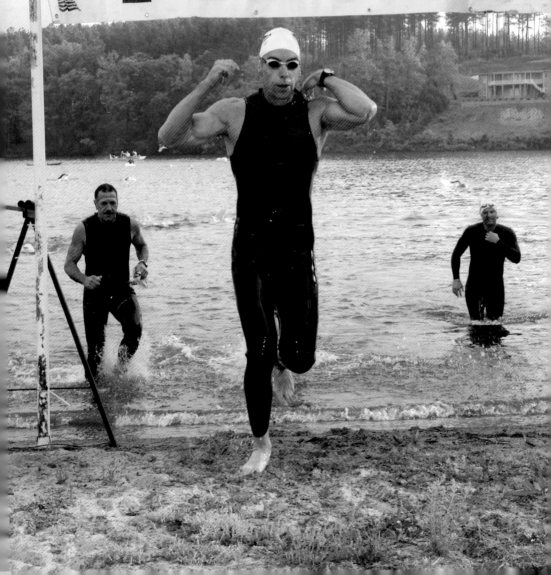

PREFACE

This is a book I wish someone had given me as a masters athlete many years ago, when I was ready to make the move from my enthusiastic 'good beginner' level to a more serious approach to triathlon. It is easy to read with a lot of tips and interesting information that would normally take a couple of years to learn yourself by trial and error.

That said, a word about what this book is not. It is not a book for the new athlete, fresh off the couch, who is still figuring out how to motivate themselves for 30 minutes of exercise a day. It is also not directed at the beginner triathlon enthusiast, new to the three-discipline sport, who is still coming to grips with the challenges of swimming, cycling and running, all right after each other.

In fact, this book assumes the reader has at least some experience in triathlon and the disciplines of swimming, cycling and running. Consequently, it does not tell the reader how to swim, cycle or run.

Instead, this book is primarily targeted at two demographics (although multiple demographics will find it useful). The first demographic is those 'good beginner' triathletes that have tasted the fun of triathlon, perhaps who have a couple of sprint triathlons under their belt, and who now want to make the commitment to a more serious approach to the sport. In essence, I wrote this book for people who want to move from the good beginner level to the intermediate level.

The second demographic is masters athletes – anyone over the age of 40, and especially over the age of 50. Some human physiology begins to change by the age of 40, but changes really take hold over 50. Moving from the good beginner triathlete level to the intermediate level is much the same no matter what the age. However, masters athletes have to confront some constraints and problems unique to age, many of which are addressed in this book.

It is written in a straightforward, conversational way that requires the minimum of effort to follow. So many triathlon- and endurance-related books are impossibly dry and hard to read in anything other than small doses.

In short, I would have written it for me, although it is over ten years too late. So, instead, I wrote it for people like me – masters athletes that see the challenge and fun in the sport, but need a short cut to some triathlon knowledge. As a result, the book is compiled from a lot of research, from talking to a lot of triathletes, and from personal triathlon experience.

Ian Stokell

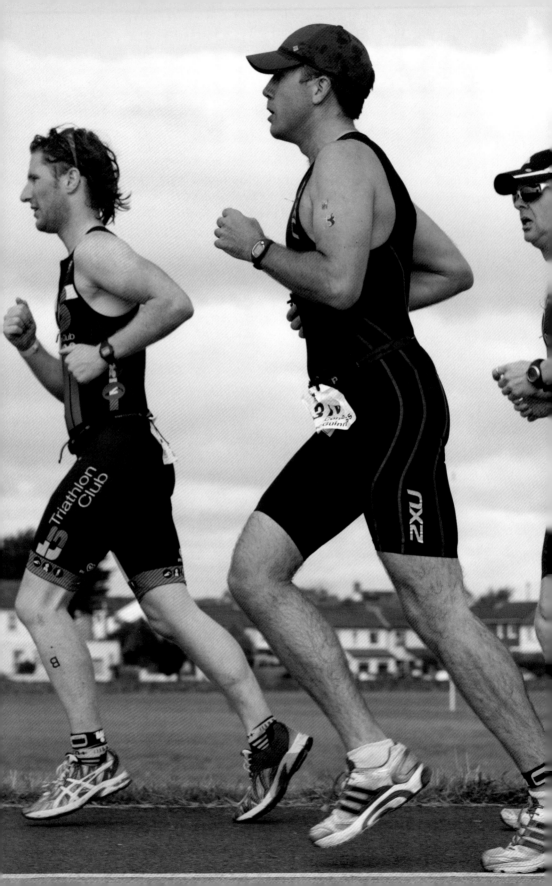

PART ONE

THE PRACTICALITIES OF TRIATHLON FOR MASTERS ATHLETES

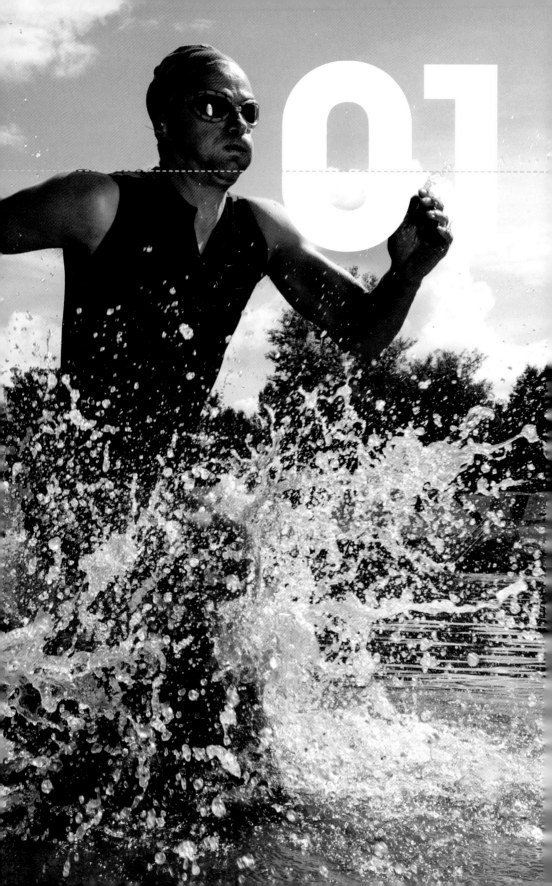

THE DIFFERENCE AGE MAKES

THREE MASTERS CONSIDERATIONS DISCUSSED IN THIS CHAPTER:

- VO$_2$ max, muscle and bone mass, fast-twitch muscles and flexibility all decline with age if left unaddressed.
- Masters athletes require more recovery time and sleep than their younger counterparts.
- High-intensity exercise and resistance training reverses most of the body's physical declines.

Many see the main focus of triathlon training as being on efficiency and endurance. The question is, from a masters athlete's perspective, how much influence does age have on performance? While physical decline is often limited up to the age of 40, there will tend to be a steeper decline after that point and certainly after 50.

Changes in body composition contribute to the common fitness declines of aging. These include increased body fat, but at the same time a loss of both muscle mass and bone mass. Some of the casualties of age also include strength, flexibility and tendon elasticity, as well as top-end speed.

The aging process affects everyone in different ways, depending on myriad factors, from genetics to injury history, fitness level to lifestyle, current weight to having a positive mental attitude.

That said, there are a number of age-related issues that can be identified as common to all athletes as they age, and which affect them to varying degrees. What follow are ten such issues, all of which will be discussed at greater length elsewhere in the book.

COMMON AGE-RELATED ISSUES FOR ATHLETICS

VO_2 max decline

VO_2 max – essentially, the amount of oxygen that can be utilised by a person during athletic activity to produce energy – declines with age, and there is nothing anyone can do to actually stop it. Some estimates put that decline as high as 1 per cent a year after one's mid-thirties. However, a lot can be done to slow down that decline. The answer is proactive, high-intensity workouts. For example, run workout sessions involving short, high-intensity interval training ranging from 30 seconds to 3 minutes, depending on fitness, with short, ever-decreasing recovery periods.

Muscle mass decline

Humans begin losing muscle mass as young as 30 years of age. By the time they reach their 50s and 60s, they are losing muscle mass at a rate of 10 per cent per decade, and even higher after 70. Proactively taking steps to increase muscle mass in older athletes helps prevent injuries by adding strength to the body, which allows for the execution of correct technique over longer periods (among other things), and in absorbing repetitive impacts – as a result of running, for example.

Resistance training can prevent muscle loss and enhance satellite cells, which will in turn allow for the rebuilding of muscles. A training programme utilising high-intensity, multi-joint lifting will benefit the body the most. In addition, increased protein in the daily diet of masters athletes will invariably help increase muscle mass when coupled with proactive resistance and high-intensity training.

Bone mass decline

Bone mass declines after the age of 40. Osteoporosis – where bones become denser and more porous, and therefore are more at risk of breaking – affects one in three women, and one in five men. Exercise can maintain bone, and in some cases build it, essentially preventing or delaying the onset of osteoporosis.

However, exercise on its own does not prevent bone loss. It also requires the correct nutrition – such as calcium and vitamin D, among others. Strength training and high-impact exercise (such as running) are most effective at building bone mass, but also the most risky, especially in masters athletes, because of the susceptibility of the body to injury as it gets older. Exercise also has to be tailored specifically to the area where the bone mass needs to be increased.

Fast-twitch muscle decline

Simply put, the body contains fast-twitch and slow-twitch muscle fibres. Fast-twitch muscle fibres contract quickly and utilise anaerobic metabolism to create fuel. Consequently, they are responsible for reaction times, explosive power and short-burst activities. However, they tire easily and consume lots

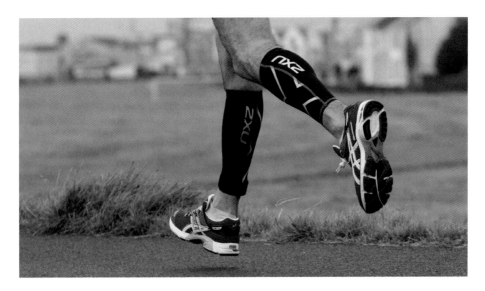

of energy. By contrast, slow-twitch muscle fibres contract slowly and utilise oxygen better, and as a result they are utilised for endurance activities such as triathlons and marathons because they fatigue at a slower rate.

Fast-twitch muscle fibres decline with age, which is why reaction times slow down as you get older, along with top-end sprinting speed and explosive movements. More accurately, fast-twitch muscles will atrophy – shrink away – without proactive, high-intensity training. So, as with many other facets of bodily decline mentioned in this chapter, fast-twitch muscle fibre decline can be slowed down with specific exercise.

Increased risk of injury

There is a much higher risk of injury as athletes age, due in no small part to the body's natural tendencies to become, for example, less flexible and increasingly fatigued with exercise. Recovery time and sleep need to be increased with age. Without that extra recovery, additional stress and fatigue is placed on older bodies, which increases the risk of injury.

Decreasing the repetitive impact on the body (such as on the bones in feet and joints) can help reduce injuries, as can implementing more focused low-impact training.

Chronic overuse injuries are the most common injuries in masters athletes, with some sources maintaining that they account for as much as 70 per cent of injuries in athletes aged 60 years of age and older.

Lack of flexibility

As the body ages it becomes less flexible in everything from joints to muscles, as well as in soft tissue generally. Lack of flexibility is one of the primary causes of injury in the older population, whether they are athletes or not. A structured programme designed to maintain flexibility needs to be integrated into every masters' training schedule. In addition, for masters athletes, nutrition can also play a large role in protecting joints from age-related damage.

Such a programme can be achieved by including yoga and plenty of stretching. This can also include increased amounts of stretching in a triathlete's warm-up and cool-down, along with stopping to stretch at an appropriate time during a workout whenever necessary.

In addition, joints not only become less flexible with age, but also lose much of their range of motion if the body is allowed to become sedentary.

Declining elasticity

Soft tissue damage is common in older athletes because ligaments, which connect joints together, and tendons, which attach muscles to bone, lose their elasticity. As a result, they are more likely to tear if they are not handled with care. This can happen without ample warming up and cooling down, and with the lack of correct technique.

Lactate threshold decline

Lactic acid builds up in your body as you train. The body does a good job of removing it, but eventually it reaches the point where it is no longer able to remove it on its own. That point is your lactate threshold, where the muscles become extremely inefficient in their oxygen use. A high threshold allows an athlete to engage in high-intensity workouts without feeling the effects of the lactic acid. However, an athlete's lactate threshold declines with age.

More recovery time and extra sleep

The simple fact is that a body requires greater recovery time as it ages. That might apply to recovery during workouts or the addition of an extra day of rest during the regular training week. The optimum time for regenerative recovery is while the body sleeps. Increased sleep for masters athletes, especially after a hard workout or race, will help the body recover and come back stronger.

The younger a triathlete, the more they hate recovery; and yet the older the triathlete, the more they love it! Recovery is a vital part of performance improvement in triathlon. Increasing recovery time will allow a triathlete to train injury-free for longer and help mentally with motivation for upcoming harder workouts.

Increased need for high-intensity and resistance training

Declines in VO_2 max, muscle mass and bone mass, lactate threshold, strength and power in masters athletes can all be slowed, and even halted altogether, with regular high-intensity workouts and resistance training. Once or twice a week,

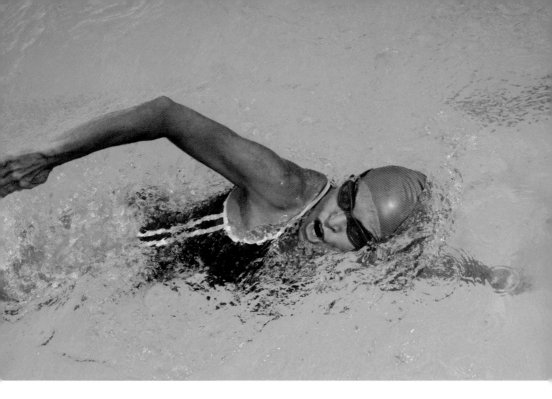

a high-intensity workout, such as interval training in the pool or on a running track, or hill repeats on the bike, should be scheduled in. Care must be taken for masters athletes, though, as high intensity workouts inevitably involve increased stresses on the body, which increase the risk of injury. The day following a high-intensity workout should be either a rest day or an easy day with low-impact training, such as a low-intensity and low-volume bike ride, or easy swim.

CONCLUSION

It should come as little surprise that many physical aspects of the body decline with age. However, much of that decline can be slowed considerably, and even halted, with regular high-intensity workouts and resistance training.

What's more, some aspects of physiology barely decline at all until much later in life. For example, endurance in a fit athlete declines just 4 per cent before the age of 55. Power and strength, however, decline much quicker, in large part due to muscle mass loss.

Even for non-athletes, remaining active, and keeping flexibility in the joints, muscles and other soft tissue, can add to both longevity and quality of life.

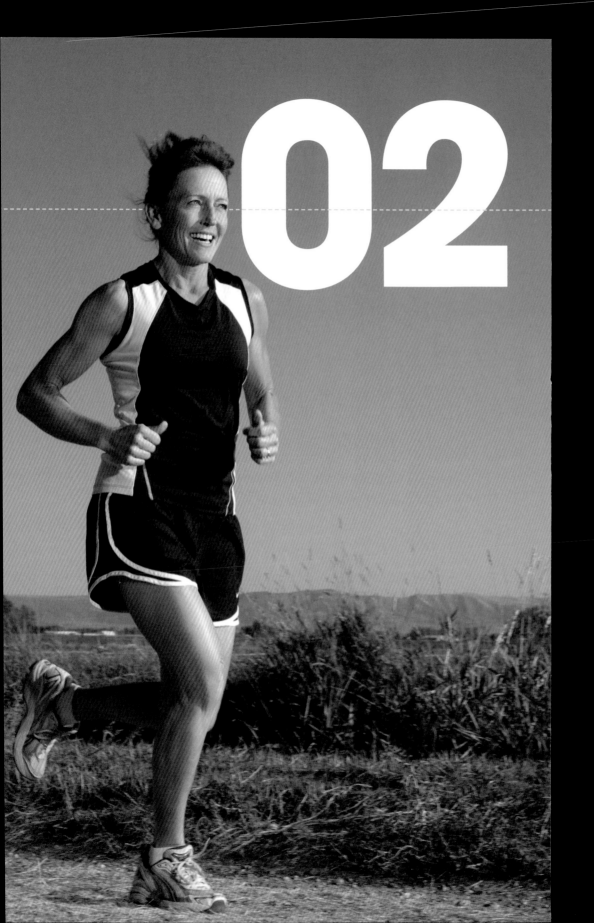

02

A LIFESTYLE COMMITMENT

**THREE MASTERS CONSIDERATIONS
DISCUSSED IN THIS CHAPTER:**

- There needs to be balance in life – everything from triathlon training and nutrition to family, friends and social activities. Stress and bad time management have a negative impact on performance.

- Gains in triathlon performance are incremental. There are no quick fixes. Training is not a sprint – it is a long-term commitment to improvement by hard work. Your lifestyle should reflect that patient pursuit of excellence.

- The older a triathlete gets, the more important sleep and recovery become to performance gains. Take a step back, sleep more, and embrace time away from the sport.

The transition from beginner triathlete – someone who dabbles in the triple-discipline art a few hours a week – to a more serious athlete with measurable performance goals and season-long training schedules is much more than simply increasing training by a few hours each week.

This chapter explores the changes that need to be addressed for any triathlete thinking of committing to a more serious pursuit of triathlon and the increased demands that will have to be addressed.

TRIATHLON IS NOT A HOBBY

Triathlon is not a hobby; it's a lifestyle. Serious triathlon training cannot be divorced from the rest of your life. So much time and energy is required to train for a sport with so many interlocking elements – from hydration to calorie intake, from time management to ensuring enough sleep and rest, from the time commitment required for actual training to expenses for equipment and travel – that anyone thinking of committing to the sport needs to stop and seriously consider if it is something they are willing to take on.

GAINS ARE INCREMENTAL

Just as triathlon gains are incremental, so they are also long-term.

There is no quick fix. For older athletes, that mantra is even more important. Slow and steady progress reduces the risk of injuries. Just as gains are expected to be incremental, so will be the extra stresses and strains that are placed on the aging body. Those increasing stresses and strains that come from longer training sessions and higher intensities need to be kept under control and managed.

The body is broken down in training, only to be strengthened again in recovery. However, that breaking down of the body has to be controlled for it to be safe.

Above all, your commitment to the triathlon lifestyle has to be sustainable and, ultimately, enjoyable. If you are not enjoying it, then why are you doing it? There are easier ways to get fit and stay healthy.

In addition, that same patient, incremental approach to performance progress has to be supported by a mental attitude that is in sync with the same long-term goals. Just as your training schedules should not expect fast returns and quick fixes, so your lifestyle commitment to triathlon should reflect that lasting, long-term outlook.

BALANCE

Because the commitment to triathlon is a lifestyle choice with incremental gains, and not a quick fix that can be completed with a speedy 2-month programme, it has to be tempered with balance. Balance is necessary in life and in triathlon. Triathlon should not, and cannot, consume your life. Triathlon training should complement your life, not control it. It should ultimately enhance all the other aspects of your life – family, friends, social life, work and career.

In addition, executed correctly, triathlon can be a very effective stress reliever (as can other endurance sports such as marathon running). The triathlon lifestyle, then, should alleviate stress, not add to it.

Importantly, a realistic appraisal should be made of your goals and desires for triathlon so that they fit in with all the other aspects of your life. That is why the importance of a realistic and achievable set of goals is fundamental to the triathlon lifestyle, along with a strategy to achieve them and a complementary training schedule based around those goals.

Realistic goals and an ongoing training schedule should be looked upon as tools to not only improve personal triathlon performance and health generally, but also bring balance into your life as you make the transition to a triathlon-oriented lifestyle.

CALORIES

First, a word about calories and the need to consume a certain amount each day. This will be repeated in more detail later in the book (see p. 82). Your body is a finely tuned engine. However, for that engine to operate correctly it requires fuel. Not just any fuel, but the right type of fuel. If the body does not get sufficient fuel (i.e. calories), it will not have enough energy to continue training at a high level.

Let's do some maths! As a general rule of thumb, in terms of calorie intake, a person needs fourteen times their bodyweight in pounds to maintain their weight. Let's take me as an example. At 6 feet 3 inches and 200 pounds, I need to consume about 2,800 calories each day (14×200) to maintain my weight. I probably burn 500–600 calories an hour in triathlon training. If I average 2 hours of training a day ($2 \times 500{-}600 = 1{,}000{-}1{,}200$ calories burned), I need to consume another 1,000–1,200 calories a day, on top of my 2,800 calories, just to maintain my weight. That is 3,800–4,000 calories a day just to maintain my current weight.

The problem for anyone involved in ongoing triathlon training is that if you do not consume enough calories, the next day or so, the body will tire and you will feel drained, tired and sapped of energy. When the body trains while tired, the likelihood of injury increases.

Personally, I feel the impact of insufficient calories the very next day. Two or three consecutive days with insufficient calories and I feel exhausted. This is not unusual.

You have to consume enough calories each day or your triathlon training will suffer and, consequently, you will feel tired and lacking energy in all other areas of your life. Being tired will lead to loss of concentration and motivation, and to a reduction of correct athletic technique, which will increase the chance of injury.

If losing weight is one of your goals, then, just like triathlon training, the change needs to be incremental. A weight loss rule of thumb is to get within 500 calories of your daily calorie intake goal. Any more than a 500-calorie deficiency will result in extreme fatigue. Weight loss, just like triathlon training, needs to be realistic and sustainable. There are no quick fixes for weight loss, especially if you want to maintain quality triathlon training while you try to shed some pounds.

NUTRITION

You should aim for a balanced approach to training as well as a balanced approach to your diet.

As mentioned above, it is not just a question of calories, but the right kind of calories. That is where nutrition management comes in. The first rule is to get enough calories. The second rule is to get the right kind of calories. You would not put diesel into a petrol engine, would you?

Chapter 9 (pages 77–85) goes into the fine detail about nutrition. For now, suffice it to say that, just as you have to reach a balance between commitment to triathlon training and all the other areas of your life, so you need balance in your diet.

Those on a vegetarian diet will face their own particular challenges to provide enough calories, and the right kind of calories, to sustain year-round triathlon training. Most age-group triathletes are pressed for time as it is, without having to become a full-time chef in order to provide enough calories and nutrition in their diet. However, even if you don't have time to prepare your own meals from scratch using vegetarian staples such as beans and lentils to maintain a sufficient protein intake, there are now a wide range of convenient (and appetising!) high-protein, low-fat meat substitutes available from most supermarkets and health food shops.

In fact, there is nothing to stop anyone tailoring their own dietary requirements to the needs of triathlon training, so read Chapter 9 and carefully evaluate your current food habits before deciding on a balanced diet that will complement your new healthy lifestyle.

SLEEP

It is hard to believe that, even in the 21st century, where we can steer cameras through the rings of Saturn and piece together injured people like the Six Million Dollar Man, we still haven't figured out how to get more than 24 hours into a day. Come on science, catch up with popular demand!

Well, we can't. And, like it or not, that means at least 6–7 hours of those 24 have to be taken up with sleep. I hear what you're saying: 'I only need 4 hours of sleep a night.' Maybe so, if your idea of exercise is to walk to your garage, get in the car and drive everywhere. However, if you intend to train for triathlon, improve your personal performance in the sport, and not crash and burn in just a few weeks, 4 hours of sleep a night is not going to cut it.

Triathlon performance improves by pushing a body to its limits, and then giving it enough time to replenish and rebuild after the damage that has just been done to it, in order to get stronger. If you cut corners on recovery time, your body will not just fail to get stronger, it could actually get weaker. That can lead to overtraining, burnout, unnecessary physical and mental stress, and ultimately injuries, especially if you are a masters athlete.

Sleep is one of the most important aspects of recovery. If you scrimp on sleep, you are not giving your body the necessary time to rebuild. In addition, the older you get, the more important sleep becomes to effective recovery.

One tip for masters triathletes and older is to add an hour or two to your night's sleep when you are in a recovery phase, especially directly following a race. Your body is going to need all the help it can get to return to full fitness.

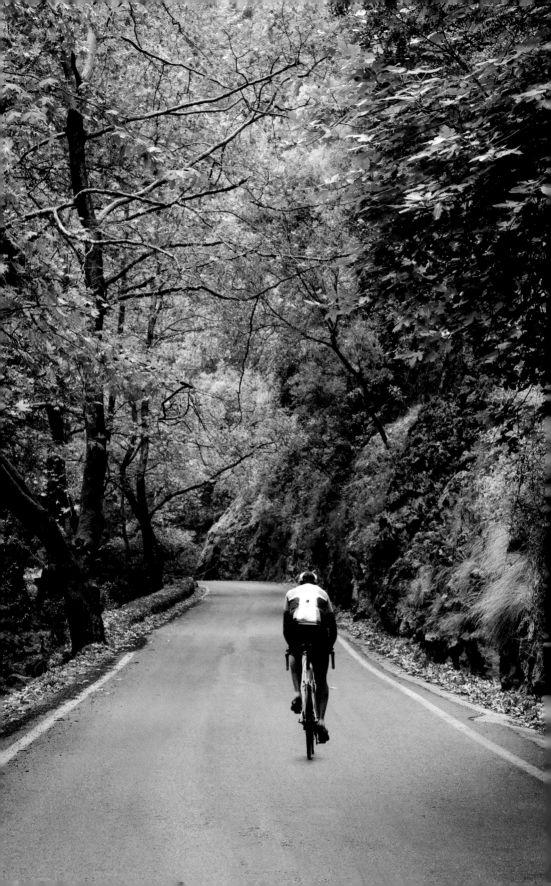

TIME MANAGEMENT

Most triathletes are 'type A' people, meaning that they always have something going on, and there are never enough hours in the day. The older they get, the more they have going on. Usually this is because they are successful in what they do, especially in business or their career. Very often, a factor contributing to their success is the ability to manage their time effectively, so they can fit everything in. Often, though, the discipline of triathlon, and the resulting fallout into the rest of their life, will come as a bit of a shock to the system.

If you hope to be successful in triathlon and avoid letting the long training time commitments negatively affect your life, you will need to become proficient in time management. If you are proficient already, fitting in the extra training hours should be a breeze. If you are not, and are used to a more laissez-faire attitude to daily scheduling, prepare for an attitude adjustment!

Reality check: an unorganised or 'go-with-the-flow' approach does not equate to less stress. Always being in a rush because you have not managed your time and commitments effectively is stressful. Reduce that stress by having a time management strategy. You are going to have to have a pre-planned training schedule and training strategy anyway, so why not have one for the rest of your busy life?

Effective time management is not simply a luxury reserved for the committed triathlete. It is a vital component in your triathlon arsenal. A little bit of planning will reduce stress and maximise available time in order to allow you to fit in all the things you want to do.

TRAINING TIME COMMITMENT

While we are discussing lifestyle changes and time management, it is worth mentioning the many hours per week that will be required by your training schedule.

If you are coming to triathlon from a single sport such as running, you will know the time commitment required to advance past the beginner stage of an endurance sport, whether you are a seasoned veteran or a weekend warrior. Multiply that by three, and then you are at the starting point for triathlon training!

If you are taking the plunge into triathlon as your first truly organised sport, you have to make sure all the training that is going to be required can fit into your weekly life and work schedule.

The time commitment to your training schedule is really the first true test of how serious you are about triathlon. Once you are on the triathlon treadmill, with self-perpetuating expectations of performance improvements and subsequent races, that time commitment does not get any less. In actuality, it will increase along with your personal commitment to improvement and more elaborate, harder-to-achieve goals.

Of course, 'more' is not necessarily 'better'. Quality of training is often just as important as quantity of training. However, even moderate personal success at a short sprint triathlon race is going to require many hard hours of physical training, and also mental training.

MEDICAL INSURANCE FOR MASTERS

For athletes over 40 – and especially for those over 50, whose bodies will demand additional recovery time and who must realistically expect to get more injuries than their 20-year-old counterparts – medical healthcare insurance will be of particular importance. UK residents reliant on the National Health Service may feel this is something they need not worry about, but bear in mind that many events take place overseas, and as your commitment to triathlon increases so may the likelihood of travel abroad.

How are you going to pay for that worse-case scenario of a torn hamstring from sprinting too hard in your run training, or a broken collarbone from a bike crash? It is an often-repeated axiom in triathlon that it is not *if* you are going to get injured, but *when*. For masters athletes especially, medical expenses are something that need to be considered sooner rather than later.

CONCLUSION

Triathlon is a lifestyle commitment. The reality is that becoming a more serious triathlete will almost certainly require at least a modicum of lifestyle change for everyone in the sport. This can have even greater significance for masters and older athletes because of the likelihood of increased general life commitments that typically come with age and success.

Time commitment to training, getting organised, paying attention to your diet and calorie intake, coping with injuries, figuring out expenses and travel – these are just some of the factors that will need to be addressed.

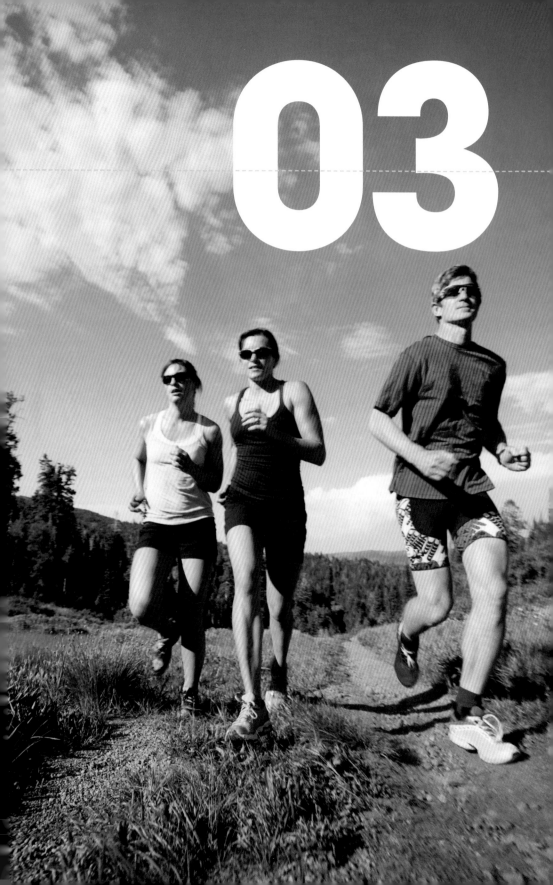

03

ESTABLISHING A SUPPORT NETWORK

> **THREE MASTERS CONSIDERATIONS DISCUSSED IN THIS CHAPTER:**
>
> - Family and friends are the foundation of any support network. The older a triathlete gets, the more important social support becomes.
>
> - A personal coach providing both highly customised training schedules and technique instruction are essential for both performance gains and to reduce the risk of injury.
>
> - Training partners are often the difference between completing the necessary training and not. Sports clubs and masters swim sessions at the local pool provide invaluable support.

For those who have been involved in regular athletic activities all their lives, a support network will likely already be in place. However, for many who are entering an athletic lifestyle over the age of 40, the expectations of both the triathlete and their friends and loved ones will be akin to exploring unknown territory.

Triathlon, especially the longer distances such as half-Ironman and full Ironman, is the epitome (or pinnacle!) of solitary sports: hour after hour of just you and the race course. It is one of the sport's true ironies, then, that you increase your chances of success by establishing a solid support network foundation in training on which you can build your triathlon dreams.

Such a support network should include resources relating to both the sport – with physical and technical instruction and advice relating to improving performance – and from a personal perspective, in terms of emotional, physical and mental well-being.

Indeed, for many masters triathletes, the prospect of finding a new circle of like-minded friends and fellow athletes becomes a large driving force behind their new-found commitment to the sport.

KEY FACTORS IN ESTABLISHING A SUPPORT NETWORK

Family and friends

The foundation for any triathlete's support network has to be family and friends. The time and effort commitments to a triathlon lifestyle are so great that immediate family have to be on-board for it to have any chance of lasting success and not be the source of animosity and resentment. Great care must be taken to be flexible and to work around family time and obligations. Family should be the foundation of your support network, and not become something that will ultimately undermine all the hard training that will have taken place.

It is often true that, for most triathletes, the older they get, the greater the family commitments. Masters-age triathletes who have families and children are likely to feel the strain between family commitments and triathlon training the most. This tends to tail off as triathletes reach 50 years of age, and children enter high school and become more independent.

Friends, especially if they are health-conscious, athletically inclined or active in a sport, can be a tremendous source of encouragement and support. Their input and interest is something that can prove invaluable in the long term.

Sometimes, however, friends – especially those who are not health-conscious, and for reasons often unrelated to you at all – will feel the need to show little support or be quick to criticise. Perhaps your proactive move towards a healthy lifestyle shows them up in a bad light or causes them to question their own unhealthy lifestyle. The harsh reality, though, is that unsupportive and negative friends should not, and probably will not, stay in your inner circle for long. A positive environment is essential for the triathlon lifestyle, and friends who do not support it should not be given the opportunity to undermine your personal goals, in triathlon or in life.

Workplace support

Most triathletes could probably go through their entire triathlon lives without their workplace knowing they are involved in triathlon. Often, though, it does no harm to let your workplace know that you are a triathlete, that you are training for races, and that at least a couple of times a year you may be taking time off from work to travel and race away from home.

One major reason is that, in an increasingly health-conscious society, many companies try to offer help to health-conscious employees in the form of in-house facilities and possible financial assistance towards membership of outside facilities, such as a health club, gym or local YMCA facility. Your company may also be open to the idea of official company teams, sponsoring a one-off triathlon team, or an after-work physical activity health programme.

Additionally, if your company does not offer it already, it may be open to some sort of flexi-time. This may allow you to work out on some mornings and not have to rush to get to work by 9am.

Companies are increasingly concerned with employee retention, and recruiting the best employees from the marketplace. As a result, you never know where the agendas between corporate and an increasingly health-conscious workforce will meet.

Personal triathlon coach

For some triathletes, the mainstay of their support network will be a personal triathlon coach. Essentially, a coach will control and guide your triathlon training and upcoming season schedule. A good coach will be a motivator, a shoulder to cry on and a disciplinarian, but ultimately someone who can take your body and mould it into a triathlete capable of completing, and even competing, in triathlon races.

Ideally, your coach should know you inside and out, along with your weaknesses and your strengths, and be able to nurture and steer your triathlon alter ego through the minefield of training and racing, to come out the other side victorious and smelling of roses! They should be able to devise a workout programme, as well as a season-long training schedule, that will ultimately improve your triathlon performance and help you reach your long-term goals.

For masters athletes, it becomes increasingly important to find a coach who understands the increased stresses and strains that are placed on the older body, no matter how athletic that body may have been 20 years previously. Everyone is different in their physical and mental make-up.

Importantly, generic training and workout schedules are of little value to masters triathletes, who should work with a coach to customise a programme according to their individual physiology and injury history.

In the absence of a personal coach, a substitute needs to be the ubiquitous workout log. You will need to write down everything and anything that relates to your training and racing. In essence, the workout log becomes a virtual coach. There is no escaping the brutal truth once all the details of your training and race are written down on paper. A good personal triathlon coach can never be replaced, of course, but necessity or otherwise may demand something less physical. In the absence of a personal coach, a detailed ongoing workout log is a must.

Training schedule

In a strange but useful way, your personalised training schedule becomes part of your support group. You consult this schedule every day and endeavour to meet its increasingly rigorous demands. As such, a well-thought-out and personalised training schedule is vital if you wish to see improvement in your triathlon performance.

Normally, your personal triathlon coach will set your schedule, taking into account your season goals as well as your likes and dislikes. The coach will also be available to rewrite the schedule at a moment's notice should the situation, or injury, dictate.

In the absence of such a personal coach, though, if someone well-versed in triathlon training schedules can write yours remotely or online, that is better than nothing at all, and, unless you are an experienced triathlete, probably better than doing it yourself.

Your training schedule is the glue that holds all your season goals and training together. Training peaks along with key 'A' races throughout the season, and goes hand-in-hand with personal and triathlon goals. As a result, the importance of a well-thought-out training schedule cannot be overestimated.

Someone to teach proper technique

In triathlon, technique is everything. Everything, that is, except physical fitness and a positive mental attitude!

However, with triathlon, especially with the longer distances, optimum technique equates to maximum efficiency. Maximum efficiency means less effort. Less effort means the ability to go longer and harder with lower energy expenditure and reduced risk of injury. Triathlon is all about physical fitness, of course, but the real key to success is technique.

As a result, one of the foundation legs of a triathlon support network has to be someone who can teach correct technique, and who can continue to evaluate that technique and improve upon it on an ongoing basis throughout the year.

That role is usually taken by a personal triathlon coach, or possibly a specialised single-discipline coach. In the absence of a coach, however, you need to find an environment where you can find correct technique being practiced and also taught. The most likely place for both is with local clubs for any of the three disciplines – swimming, cycling, running – or a local triathlon club, or gym.

Local clubs will always have athletes participating who will offer technique pointers. In addition, local clubs will have designated sessions throughout the week that will be coached and monitored. Once you have joined the club, these sessions will probably be free to members, or available for a small fee. They also provide a ready-made pool of training partners.

Training partners

Triathlon is a very solitary sport in many regards, often with long hours alone with your thoughts in both training and in races. That said, training partners can provide much-needed companionship in the long days and weeks of training.

They can also be a source of motivation just to get out of bed in the early morning to train, never mind keeping you to your schedule or attaining your triathlon goals. Knowing someone else is next to you going through the same experience can be comforting as you start out on a rainy ride when it is barely dawn.

An ideal scenario would be to team up with someone who is planning to do the same upcoming 'A' race as you, especially if you share roughly the same level of fitness. Not only can you combine training sessions and resources, but you might even be able to pool travel expenses and share costs for the race itself.

Of course, you can have, and probably will have, multiple training partners for the different disciplines in addition to ones that change from week to week. They may not even be triathletes, but instead focused on a single sport.

A training partner should be low-maintenance and dependable! There is nothing worse than having to brave the early morning winter weather to get to the start of a long ride only to have to wait 20 minutes because your training partner hit the snooze button earlier or had not prepared their equipment or nutrition the night before and had to rush to get it completed the morning of the ride. Someone with considerable commitments outside of training – such as family or work – may also not be the best training partner, except for the occasional session.

In training, you need to eliminate the reasons for not training. Make no mistake, you will come up with plenty of reasons yourself why you should not do tomorrow's training session, so the last thing you need is a high-maintenance training partner providing you with more.

TRAINING FACILITIES AND SUPPORT
Local masters swim sessions
As mentioned previously, technique is important in all three triathlon disciplines. However, the one that is most affected by technique is swimming. Good technique in swimming is essential for energy-saving efficiency and speed through the water. Bad swimming technique may well put an end to your triathlon in the second half of the race.

Your local pool, for example, will almost certainly offer masters swimming sessions a few times a week. They will meet at various times, and each session will be taught by a designated coach.

Such sessions are good for discipline and technique, as well as providing a social outlet where you can converse with like-minded individuals. They will probably feature coached swim drills, which are important for technique and swim stamina. You may not have access to swim drills elsewhere, especially if you do not have a coach, or if your triathlon coach does not have a background or expertise in swimming.

Because multiple coaches are involved in the sessions, each with their own coaching style and level of competency, it is a good idea to attend a number of sessions and determine which coaches are well matched with your preferred coaching likes and dislikes.

Local swim/bike/run clubs

Local swim/bike/running/triathlon/athletics clubs are always a good resource, and collectively offer a vast variety of options. Aside from the masters swimming sessions at the local pool, as mentioned above, you can also probably find open water swimming sessions through the local triathlon club, interval training and speed work at the local running track through an athletics club, group bike rides courtesy of the local cycling club, or group running sessions where you can usually be matched up with runners of a similar ability running at a similar miles-per-minute pace.

As with any local club, you will probably find them full of members willing to pool their own resources and contacts in an effort to help other members. Networking prospects and contacts abound, and can often lead to individual training partners, medical advice, perhaps even business and travel opportunities.

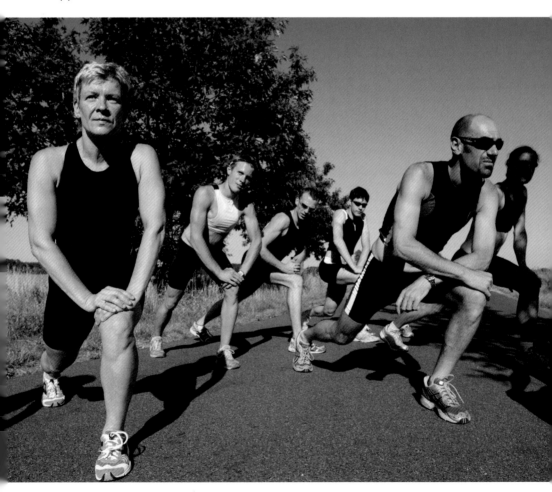

Local gym

Strength training plays a major role in triathlon training, not just for the professionals, but for masters athletes as well.

Strength and weight training are especially vital to newer triathletes that do not have all round or specific strength fitness to maintain correct technique for long periods of time. If you don't have the strength to maintain correct technique, you will eventually lapse into bad technique. And when you start practising bad technique, you put stresses and strains on your body that increase risk of injury. This is especially true for older athletes.

Strength training is essential for every triathlete, but especially masters triathletes, because of the deteriorating muscle and bone mass described earlier.

A great addition to a support network is the local gym. Membership is money well spent, and relatively cheap, as it allows you to use the weight-training facilities, plus the pool, as well as treadmills, and hot tubs and saunas for tired muscles.

Any triathlete will need access to some sort of gym for their training schedule. The great thing about a local commercial gym is that you will usually find in-house trainers on hand to give sage advice about technique and even exercise selection. However, that is not always the case with some local gyms, where you are more likely to be left to your own devices.

Your personal coach will probably be selecting weight-lifting and strength exercises for your training schedule, so the lack of in-house gym trainers at your local gym may not be an issue, as long as your personal coach can also show you correct technique. And there will probably be no shortage of other gym users to spot you for lifting heavy weights or to give you advice, whether you want it or not!

PERSONAL MENTOR

As in any industry or profession, having a personal mentor can be invaluable. The resources that a mentor can bring to bear can be the difference between success and failure.

Triathlon is no different. If you can find a personal mentor who is more experienced than yourself, and essentially better at the sport than you are, it can save you months and possibly years of trial and error and wasted effort. The best way to find a mentor is through a recommendation from someone you know or word of mouth. Your local triathlon club will have triathletes of varying levels that may be only too willing to share their experience and knowledge. Having someone in your support network who has already travelled much of the road you are about to travel can also bring considerable fun to the table, allowing you to enjoy the correct path without having to suffer long and often painful periods of experimentation.

A personal mentor is much more than a coach. They are there as a resource in all things triathlon. One of the things they can advise you on is obtaining a coach, or, if a coach is already on-board, if they are the right coach for you. For example, not all coaches are created equal, not just in terms of knowledge and experience, but in style as well. They may not be a good fit for you, and it may take a third party to help you recognise that.

A personal mentor is someone you can turn to for advice, and whose experience and resources will be able to guide you through the often-difficult times of the triathlon lifestyle, with all its complexities and demands.

ONLINE SUPPORT
Social media

We are all children of our time, whether we like it or not. Fifteen years or so ago, the very notion of online chat consisted of barely interactive text-based bulletin board services. Now, though, social media is pervasive, and it seems that everyone is on Facebook and has their own Twitter account.

Social media are intended to be interactive. For the most part, they are also designed to allow you to find and develop relationships with like-minded people.

Because the very definition of social media is to be social and interactive, people are only too willing to share their knowledge. Actively 'friending' and 'following' other like-minded people on the various social media services can quickly build up into a considerable online resource.

In addition, these online resources and virtual friends can often progress into the acquisition of training partners and useful resources in the real world.

As ever, the key concern is to enjoy your interactions, and especially to avoid letting them create any stress or confusion. Keep a critical attitude to the wealth of information that's available, and take care not to let anything disrupt any regime you have in place unless you feel sure you want to incorporate it into your programme.

Online forums and interactive reader responses

In addition to social media such as Facebook and Twitter, there are numerous online forums aimed at every subject and sport imaginable. These can provide extremely useful information, and although it sometimes seems that some of those who frequent such virtual meeting places do so simply to hear themselves talk, there are many knowledgeable and accommodating participants that are only too willing to share what they know.

Many of these forums also have regular participants and use the resource as a virtual meeting place, exchanging ideas and training tips. You can get to know many of the participants on more than an occasional basis, building up long-term friendships and adding another piece to your support network.

Another place for information and interactive advice is with reader responses that often follow articles posted online and on websites. Most magazines online feature an interactive facility directly following an article where readers can comment on the article, add their own viewpoint on the subject and reply to other reader comments. While this is not as formal as either social media or online forums, it can still be a good resource for information and interactive knowledge.

Remote networking

Whenever you go to races or attend seminars or training sessions away from home, you are going to meet people with the same interests and goals as yourself. If you hit it off with someone, be sure to get his or her contact information. The triathlete demographic is increasingly becoming one of the most social media-savvy demographics in the world. The only thing triathletes love more than doing triathlons is telling people about it and sharing the experience with social media updates and blogs.

You may end up only meeting up with these people occasionally when you travel to a race, but they will always be available online and via email, blogs, social media outlets and – dare I say something so old school – the telephone!

The important thing to remember is that your support network doesn't have to consist of people and resources that you can only access in real time and in person. In this day and age of busy schedules and 'never enough time', virtual access to people in your own time and on your own terms opens up the possibility of myriad resources that would not have been available to triathletes just a few years ago.

CONCLUSION

Establishing a comprehensive, knowledgeable and enthusiastic support network is crucial to long-term success in triathlon. It is hard, from both a physical and mental perspective, to train in isolation. Such a network provides support for your triathlon efforts, as well as motivation and fun.

For masters and older athletes, this interaction with fellow triathletes of their own age provides a much-needed social channel, offering support and encouragement. Often, for masters athletes, the social side of the sport can be as important as the personal performance enhancement goals, much more so than for their younger counterparts.

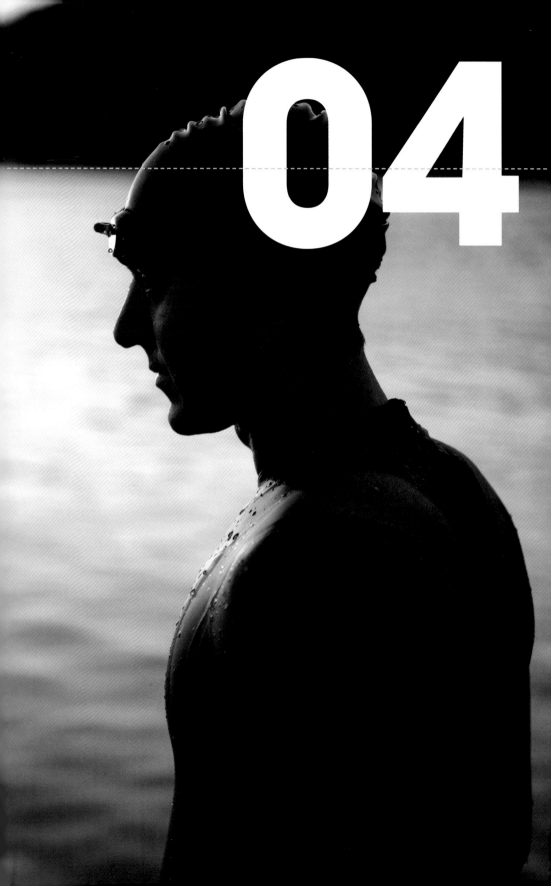

04

TRIATHLON IS A MENTAL SPORT

**THREE MASTERS CONSIDERATIONS
DISCUSSED IN THIS CHAPTER:**

- A positive mental attitude is essential, especially for masters athletes, who may find the physical and mental challenges of the long distances in triathlons harder to cope with.

- Like participation in any sport, confidence is a major key to success. Focus on your mental strength as well as physical strength, but train to improve your weakest disciplines.

- One of the most difficult mental strengths for masters athletes is to maintain flexibility and be ready to adapt to changing circumstances.

It sounds like a contradiction, but first and foremost, triathlon is a mental sport. Obtaining the required fitness for whatever is your intended race distance is a huge mental commitment. However, the mental challenge does not end there. Once adequate fitness is obtained, at any level, from beginner to professional, success in a triathlon race is predominantly the result of a positive, never-say-die, relentless mental attitude. The longer the race, the more you will be tested to your mental limits.

While there are many books on the mental complexities and intricacies of sport, this chapter focuses only on what I would consider to be the main aspects as they relate to triathlon: a positive mental attitude, flexibility, and the need to adapt to ever-changing training and race environments and circumstances in order to achieve your athletic goals.

Triathlon is a mental game and your mind has to reach the finish line before your body. Once your mind gets there, your body will follow. However, if your mind is not in the race, or the training session, your body will soon crash and burn.

There is one fundamental rule for a positive mental approach in triathlon, as well as in life: 'Do not look for excuses, look for answers.'

There are three keys to a successful mental approach in triathlon. First is a positive mental attitude. Nothing bad will come from always staying positive, whereas something bad will always ultimately result from being consistently negative. The second and third keys to success are certainly complementary, easily recognisable in their own right, and may be difficult for those older masters athletes who are set in their successful ways, but both are essential: flexibility in everything you do and the need to adapt to ever-changing circumstances.

A POSITIVE MENTAL ATTITUDE

Committing to triathlon as a way to fitness, and then competitive triathlon in the form of races, is a major undertaking. With the amount of training required just to reach the start line, there is no place for negativity. Remaining positive is not a luxury, it is a necessity. Negative thoughts are an inevitable self-fulfilling prophesy, destined for failure, while positive thoughts will lead to success.

For those who are not naturally optimists, and even for those that are, there are a number of main points to pay attention to.

Confidence – focus on your strengths

Everyone has strengths. You just have to find them.

Most people, especially age-groupers, come to triathlon from a single sport – such as swimming, biking or running. Having a dominant discipline within triathlon is certainly a benefit. A good runner can certainly take confidence from knowing that they will probably have a solid run to finish up the triathlon race with, just as a good swimmer can confidently expect to be with the front pack coming into the first transition (referred to as T1 for short).

One danger, though, is for someone who is good at running, for example, to schedule in more running than they should in their training, to the exclusion of the other disciplines. Maybe it makes them feel good to be out there running or they think it makes them look good to be at the front of a group training run. However, if anything, having a dominant single sport discipline should free up more time in your schedule to concentrate on the other two disciplines that are not as good.

Alternatively, your strengths may well not be related to an individual discipline. Maybe your strengths are related to a character trait. Perseverance may be your forte, or a willingness to learn or practise something until you improve. Being relentless in pursuit of a goal is a definite benefit for a triathlete. Actually, that is sort of mandatory.

Whatever your strengths are, find a way to leverage them into your triathlon training and racing, and know how to bring them into play when the going starts to get tough. Because if there is one certainty in triathlon, it is that the going will get tough, whether you are a beginner age-grouper or a seasoned professional.

Positive self-talk

Try to develop a habit of talking to yourself in training, as well as in races. However, if you do, keep all chatter positive. Positive self-talk can be a powerful weapon if used correctly. It allows you to focus on a single constructive facet of the current physical challenge at any one time, from 'Keep pushing up to the top of this hill' to 'Maintain this cadence' on the bike.

If you are not used to positive self-talk, simply imagine a super-positive coach standing beside you offering encouragement. What would they say to you? More importantly, as you are the coach as well as the coached in this scenario, what would you want them to say to help you through the next few minutes or few seconds? Once you have figured that out, either verbalise it externally or repeat it over and over inside your head.

However, as with all coaching advice, make sure you listen and find a way to apply the coaching advice!

Phrase everything with a positive spin

Phrasing all suggestions and constructive criticism with a positive slant is fundamental to maintaining a positive attitude. Whether it is coming from your real life coach, or your virtual 'self-talk' coach, focusing on the positive, or an optimistic view of what is required, helps instil an overall positive mental attitude and a sense of 'can do'.

For example, instead of focusing on the negative aspects of your technique, focus on what positive steps you need to immediately take to ensure good technique.

The goal is always to instil a positive culture into your training and racing, and into your personal triathlon demeanour. The mountains you will have to climb in your triathlon journey are Everest-like in their size, and the later in life you start that journey, the bigger they will appear.

You will not succeed in triathlon if all you have to offer is a negative attitude. If you are not a natural optimist, you will need to consciously adopt a positive attitude about everything – from training to injuries, hill repeats to rehab – so one of the most constructive tools you can develop from the outset is to nurture a positive mindset, even if it is consciously self-taught over the years.

Motivation and goal setting

Motivation and goal setting go hand in hand. They are both crucial to triathlon success and indispensable in developing a positive mental attitude. With motivation, figuring out why you want to train in triathlon and which races you want to compete in is not only crucial to formulating a training schedule, it is something you will probably need to revisit many times in the winter months when you have to get up at 6 am and train for hours in the rain and cold before work! So the quicker you figure it out the better for you.

Short-term, medium-term and long-term triathlon goals, and a well-thought-out and concise athletic strategy in how to achieve them, are the foundations on which all your training and upcoming racing will be based. In addition, having a step-by-step path outlined in front of you helps develop a sustainable positive mental attitude, even in the face of the inevitable triathlon setbacks. See the next chapter for more on this subject.

Task relevance

In short, this means focusing on those immediate tasks that need to be completed in order to move to the next stage of whatever it is you are doing, whether that is the immediate workout session, your training schedule or during a race.

Even though this may seem like common sense once someone points it out, for most people, this seems to be one the most difficult skills to acquire. The ability to prioritise the most important tasks first, and to accomplish them adequately before moving to the next step towards a designated goal, seems to pass most people by, whether we are talking about triathlon or life in general.

Just as important is the ability to avoid distraction. To an extent, this can be traced to what type of athlete you are. The importance of avoiding unnecessary distractions is as vital as being able to prioritise tasks in order of immediate importance.

For most people, being able to recognise the important tasks that need to be accomplished first, and to differentiate them from distractions that will prevent or delay completion of an immediate goal, is something that will take practice. In triathlon, it will come with an accumulation of training hours and race experience. A good personal coach should be able to help an athlete develop this important skill.

Develop a positive attitude during training

There is no escaping the notion that the best training for a sport is the sport itself. The best training for a running race is to run. The best training for a swimming race is swim practice in a pool or open water. The best training for cycling is to ride a bike, either out on the road, on the trails, or even on a stationary trainer.

It makes perfect sense, then, that the best way to develop a positive mental attitude, to be called upon when the chips are down and you are under race pressure, is to develop a positive mental attitude in training. If you have a positive, never-say-die mental attitude in your training, it will be an easy switch to utilise it during a race. However, if you have a negative attitude

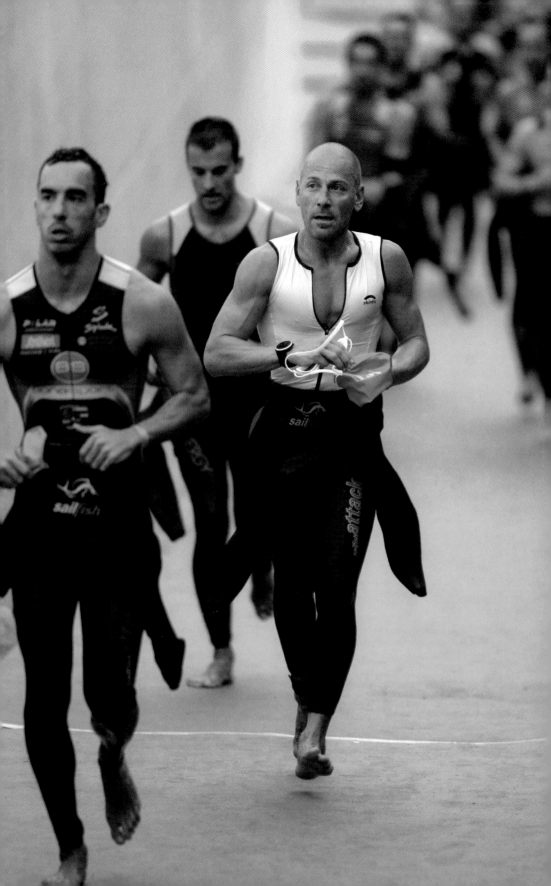

during training, where you constantly fail to complete your training schedule or individual workout session, then expecting to have a positive mental attitude during an actual race, when competitive pressure is on, is going to be a stretch.

Do not leave it to the last second, or halfway through an actual triathlon race, to figure out you do not have enough of a positive mental attitude foundation to call on for help when you need it most. Pressure in training will be magnified tenfold in an actual race.

Whatever can go wrong in a race probably will, so arm yourself against its negative impact by developing a positive mental attitude during training.

Mental imagery

Mental imagery, or 'visualisation,' has now almost become embedded in the cultural lexicon.

The fact is, though, that the visualisation technique of seeing yourself successfully accomplishing a task or goal is a powerful tool in the hands of a skilled and experienced athlete. The sooner you begin training yourself to take advantage of its motivation and positive powers the better.

In addition, visualisation is not simply a 'big picture' device where you 'see' yourself crossing the finish line successfully. It can also be applied, and is probably most effective, when used as a short-term tool to overcome immediate, but very real, obstacles.

'See' yourself climbing a steep section of the cycling course. In doing so, employ all your senses in the successful mental exercise, not just mental imagery. Try to feel your breath increasing as you climb the hill. Feel the strain on your leg muscles, the crosswind in your hair as you struggle to control the bike, and the smell of the oil you used on your gears before placing your bike in transition 2 the night before. Never mind 'Be the ball.' Instead, just visualise being yourself successfully completing the entire triathlon race course.

Also, use it in training, for bike, run and swim sessions. Train as you want to race. If you want to use visualisation techniques for your race – and let's be honest, virtually all top triathletes and professionals do – then start using them in training.

Visualisation works. However, it is a somewhat unnatural skill that takes practice and time to develop effectively and comprehensively. Begin using it as soon as you can and as often as you can, for it to be at its most effective.

Have a personal mantra

A personal mantra is a form of positive reinforcement. It can be tied to why you are doing triathlon in the first place – for example, 'I am in control of when I stop' – or it can be practical self-encouragement – for example, 'One small step at a time.'

Whatever the origin of the personal mantra, however, it is used as a motivational device that you call on during training or during a race in order to help you overcome tough times.

To repeat, in triathlon, the tough times are coming, and the more weapons you have in your arsenal to combat them the better.

FLEXIBILITY AND ADAPTING TO CHANGING CIRCUMSTANCES

Triathlon training is awash with the possibility of injuries and other setbacks due to relentlessly long and demanding training sessions, day after day, week after week. That said, a triathlete has to accept that injuries are part of the long-term training cycle.

Everyone gets injured. Usually everyone gets injured multiple times, and sometimes on a frustratingly regular basis. For masters athletes, this is especially true if you do not respect the need for adequate recovery time to be built in to your training schedule and the notion that performance gains are incremental. How you physically and mentally cope with injuries is the key to eventual triathlon success.

Flexibility in your training regime is not a luxury; it is a fundamental requirement in getting to the start line. Many triathletes have little patience with easing off the training accelerator when injuries demand that they should. However, if you do not learn patience and flexibility in training for triathlon, you will not last long in the sport. This applies to triathletes of any age, but especially to masters athletes and older, where the body inevitably demands more attention.

Triathletes faced with an injury, training-related or otherwise, really have two choices. The first is to give up triathlon and look for a less punishing way to get fit or maintain fitness. The second is to adjust their training on the fly and continue training as best they can while giving the injury time to recover.

The redeeming feature for triathlon over a single discipline sport is that once an injury has been sustained, it is often possible to continue training, at least to a point, in at least one of the other disciplines, while the damage is repaired. For example, if you sustain a calf injury it is possible to emphasise swim training in your schedule – with no leg kick, because swimming is probably 90 per cent upper body use – coupled with extra gym work using weights with the upper body, or aerobic training from a sitting position.

In such a situation, though, it is doubly important to be flexible with your goal setting – adapting and setting achievable physical and practical short-term, and if necessary medium-term, goals to get to the other side of rehab.

Other setbacks to training can be totally unrelated to triathlon and physical exercise. These can be anything from family or work commitments, to travel and scheduling conflicts. Just as in a race, you have to be completely prepared mentally, and unfazed by external factors influencing (and often trying to derail) your triathlon goals.

Other factors play a considerable part in a positive mental approach, but also in getting an athlete to focus on the demands of training. The importance of a well-thought-out training schedule and season plan gives direction to the upcoming hard work, provides a recognisable and documentable step-by-step process to personal success, and, very importantly, helps prevent burnout, both mentally and physically. As discussed in Chapter 6 (pages 51–7), attention to this goes a long way to getting an athlete's mind in the proverbial game.

The mental side of the sport does not exist in autonomy; it is directly connected to the physical. As a result, there are many other facets and tools, discussed elsewhere in this book, that can be utilised to instil and maintain a healthy mental attitude. These include everything from getting a coach that understands you as an athlete and your mental perspective, to keeping a workout log and establishing a support system, establishing exciting long-term goals, and building a solid physical foundation.

What type of person you are also plays a role in your mental approach. Are you the type of triathlete who is motivated by the achievement of success or the type of triathlete who is motivated by the avoidance of failure? While the line between the two often overlaps, someone who is motivated by the avoidance of failure will most often perform best when a task is either very hard or very easy. The triathlete who is motivated by the achievement of success tends not to look on failure as a bad thing and will do well when a task has the possibility of only a 50/50 chance of success.

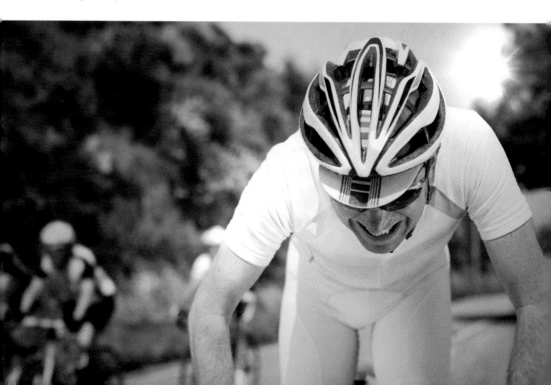

MASTERS ATHLETES SET IN THEIR WAYS

The older a triathlete gets, the more they are set in their ways and the greater the struggle to get them to change. Often it is because they are comfortable doing something a certain way, or that they know it makes them look good, or that they are not used to being accountable for such factors as poor technique.

The result is that the mental side of the sport and the need to be flexible and to adapt to ever changing training and race conditions is very often one of the hardest parts to overcome for masters triathletes. Many (typically type A, go-getter personalities) come from a successful background, often in business, and are used to taking control. While that may have worked, and still works, in many aspects of their professional life, the ability to adapt to ever-evolving circumstances, often where you do not have control, is vital to triathlon success.

CONCLUSION

Whether you are a seasoned, battle-worn masters athlete or a twenty-something convinced of your body's invincibility, mastering the mental side of the sport is a fundamental requirement for triathlon success.

A flexible, positive mindset will soon become your secret weapon, helping you with everything from advanced visualisation techniques to goal setting, from injury rehab to the alleviation of pre-race nerves.

Even for professional triathletes, in the effort to obtain a certain level of personal fitness – and certainly once that level of fitness has been achieved – the sport becomes mostly mental.

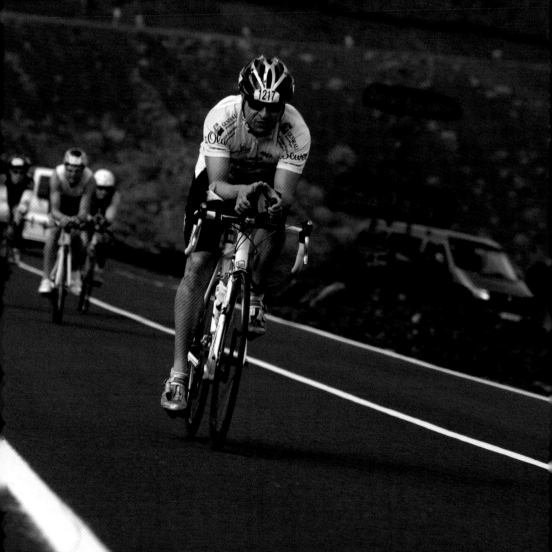

05

MOTIVATION AND GOAL SETTING

**THREE MASTERS CONSIDERATIONS
DISCUSSED IN THIS CHAPTER:**

- It is particularly important for masters athletes, who must contend with both the passage of time and memories of past glories, to set performance goals, not outcome goals.

- Goals for masters athletes must be linked to current training and competition performances.

- Future goals must be attainable. It defeats the purpose of having goals to set unobtainable goals that do not take into consideration age-specific performance declines.

There are two pressing reasons for setting goals: motivation and to provide a direction for athletic training. However, while goal setting is a fundamental motivational tool, to get motivated an athlete has to know why they are participating in the sport in the first place.

The first step in setting goals is to sit down and have a heart-to-heart with yourself. Basic questions need to be answered. Without those answers, there is no way of knowing what goals to set and, more importantly, how to establish a strategy to achieve them.

Many questions need to be asked. However, be warned: a simple question can open up a can of worms, and unleash personal unanswered questions you have been keeping under the internal lock and key for years.

For example, with regard to the question 'why are you doing triathlon?', is your initial answer to prove that you can still perform and want to challenge yourself even though you are 50 years old? That is probably not the real answer. It opens up an even bigger question that needs to be confronted. Why do you think you need to perform and challenge yourself? If you are honest with yourself, those deeper answers can get pretty uncomfortable.

The questions that should be asked are many and varied. Let's breach the dam and open the floodgates with some examples of questions: What is your understanding of the sport? How committed to the sport are you? Are you simply committed to exercise and improving your health, and not really to triathlon? Because, if you are, then there are less painful ways to keep fit!

What level do you want to reach within the sport? The higher the level, the tougher it is going to be with relentless training, day in and day out. Are you aware of the skills that need to be attained for the level you wish to compete at? Are you aware of the fitness levels? Can your body handle that amount of punishment?

Are you aware of the time commitment that triathlon requires, even for the short distances? Are you aware of the strain it can put on your social life, especially if you plan on moving up to the half-Ironman distance and beyond? Where does it fit in with your life goals? Are you aware of the costs? Travelling to races is expensive.

Triathlon goals do not exist in isolation. They are integrated with life goals, training schedules, financial constraints and non-sporting future plans.

Most triathletes will be likely to plan their training schedules and triathlon goals around two or three key 'A' races throughout a season. Those race dates will depend on personal factors and what other things are going on in your life.

However, never forget that, as the old saying goes, 'Life is what happens when you're busy making plans.'

KEY ELEMENTS IN ESTABLISHING GOALS

Types of goals

There are three types of goals:

- outcome goals
- performance goals
- process goals.

Outcome goals usually focus on the result of a competitive event – for example, winning a championship. Performance goals focus on personal standards and individual performances, such as bettering a personal best time at the mile. Process goals are actions an individual must accomplish on the way to achieving those goals. They focus on what an individual must do to perform well, such as implementing good technique.

For the most part, performance goals are better than outcome goals, even though the latter have their uses as a motivational tool away from direct competition. For the most part, though, on an ongoing basis, the negative repercussions of outcome goals far outweigh their potential benefits.

Increased anxiety and lower self-confidence in the heat of competition are common for athletes who emphasise outcome goals. Personal success is often dictated by other athletes' performances. In contrast, athletes that set performance goals, for the most part, experience the opposite to those who set outcome goals. They have less anxiety and increased self-confidence. By contrast, it is their own actions that dictate the success of their own performance goals, not other athletes' performances.

Any programme should aim for a balance between all three – performance, process and outcome goals. Practically speaking, they should be separated into short-term, medium-term and long-term goals.

Long-term goals, to no-one's surprise, are those targets that an athlete is ultimately progressing towards. Practically speaking, they are of limited use on a day-to-day training basis. However, there needs to be a strategy to achieve them. That is where medium- and short-term goals come into play.

On that pathway towards those long-term goals, think of short-term goals as those things that need to be done today or in the next training session. Perhaps they are small technique adjustments designed to help improve efficiency or reduce the possibility of injury.

Medium-term goals can be everything in between. A medium-term goal could refer to an athlete's next three-week block of training before a required week of active recovery. Or a medium-term goal could involve a race or practice race set for two months' time.

There is also a distinction made between subjective goals and objective goals. The easiest way to understand subjective goals is to envisage going out and giving it your best shot. Objective goals, by contrast, relate to personal performance. Simply put, they are definable and measurable. For example, the need to reduce running speed by 10 seconds per mile. Having a definable objective goal may then allow for the focus to be placed on specific technique improvements.

Set performance goals, not outcome goals

Wherever possible, then, avoid setting outcome goals, such as 'I am going to win the race.' The trouble with triathlon is that there are so many moving parts which contribute to the whole. For example, you are not even dealing with a single discipline; it is three disciplines over a long time period. That is not even referring to volume of training, but just race time. So many factors can influence your race. Ultimately, you need to focus only on what you can control.

What can be controlled is your own performance. Even then, you may not be able to completely control that. However, you are more likely to be able to control your own performance than someone else's. You cannot control how other athletes perform, or the environmental conditions, or race day technical problems, or bad luck, or …

Performance goals, in contrast, are concerned with how you perform. They are goals set in relation to personal standards. However, they can also be counterproductive; for example, if you are trying to compare times for a set distance, but from different race courses. Obviously, terrain and environmental conditions again play a part in timed goals.

Often it is best to work towards other performance-oriented goals, such as reducing heart rate at a given speed, or the ability to maintain road speed on the bike while keeping within a certain zone of effort.

Triathlon, and goal setting, to a great extent, are all about control and focus. You need to focus on what you personally can control, both in a competitive race and in training.

As a result, learn to differentiate between performance goals and outcome goals when goal setting, and focus more on motivating factors you can control rather than those you cannot.

Write goals down and regularly monitor progress

Goals should not remain in your head; they need to be written down. Once something is written down, it is out there in the world. Telling people your goals makes it harder to take them back.

Post a printed piece of paper with your goals on up where you can see it. Never tuck it away in a drawer. Out of sight is truly out of mind. You will miraculously find out that there are a thousand reasons why you should not train tomorrow, and only a handful of reasons why you should.

Writing down goals and keeping them visible allows them to be continually monitored. Monitoring goals is a fundamental and necessary part of goal setting. Goals need to be continually monitored, preferably by the goal setter, and not just the athlete's coach. That is in order to make sure they are being adhered to and that the agreed upon goal achievement strategy is working.

The best piece of advice I give to people that tell me they want to get fitter and have bought a treadmill/stationary bike is to place the equipment next to their bed. It is the last thing they see before they turn out the light and go to sleep, and the first thing they see when they get up in the morning. If that is not a visual reminder to achieve set goals, then I do not know what is! There is no escaping your fitness goals if the piece of equipment is nudging into your consciousness the second you open your eyes in the morning.

However, the primary rule for bedroom-located fitness equipment is not to use it as a clothes horse! 'Out of sight, out of mind' – in this case lost under a pile of dirty washing – cannot be allowed to encroach on the bedroom fitness equipment.

Set realistic and attainable goals

Probably the main reason many people give up fitness and athlete-oriented goals, especially those who are inexperienced with them, is because the goals they set are too hard to achieve or require too much of a commitment to complete. Given a myriad of different factors – from lifestyle to family to work constraints – they are simply unrealistic.

There are two main rules of goal setting. The first is that, given your current fitness level, they should be realistic in that you should think you can achieve them. Second, they should be attainable in that they are not so hard physically that you will dread upcoming training sessions and then get discouraged when you are unable to attain them.

Goals (and we are talking short- and medium-term goals here) should be hard enough to give you a sense of satisfaction when you achieve them, and not too easy that you get bored in training because they require little effort to complete.

Remember that performance improvement in triathlon is incremental. It is not a sprint after all. Improvement comes from month after month of quality and consistent training.

Everyone likes their 'comfort zone.' It is called the 'comfort zone' for a reason, after all! However, improvement in triathlon comes by pushing out of your comfort zone and challenging your body and what it is capable of doing, then taking recovery time to allow your body to rebuild, strengthen and come back stronger.

Goal setting for athletes should be specific

Goals should be specific. The vaguer you are in setting your goals, the less likely it is that you will achieve them. Alternatively, but with more drama, the more likely it is that you will fail! Depending on your personality, that may be exactly why you set vague goals. They become a self-fulfilling prophesy.

Goals should be specific, but not complex. In addition, they should be straightforward and should clearly define what is to be achieved. Instead of focusing on a grand goal, focus on a series of smaller, attainable but specific short-term goals, which incrementally progress towards the big prize.

Always remember the often-repeated training rule in triathlon is that increased performance is incremental and there are no quick fixes.

Clearly identify the time constraints

Another essential tool in the armoury of successful goal setting is to identify time constraints. It is of little use to say, 'In the next couple of years I am going to complete a half-Ironman distance race.' That is a recipe for failure.

The best way is to put yourself on the proverbial spot and hold yourself accountable for your own training and success is by signing up for a half-Ironman distance race six months away. Then plunk down your hard-earned money – let's be honest, nothing motivates faster than paying out money – and tell everyone you know that you've signed up for the race and that is why you are training. Now you have gone and done it! You have six months to not look like a fake! There is no way out of it without looking like you have bailed. Excellent!

You say, 'Sometime in the next year or so I want to be capable of a ten-mile run in training.' Lame! Instead say, 'Within the next 90 days I will have completed a ten-mile training run and not ended up in the emergency room as a result.' That's more like it! Now all you have to do is get together with your coach and figure out a training strategy to obtain that goal within the 90-day cut-off period. Write that goal in big letters on sheets of paper and pin one above your desk at work and a second one on the fridge at home.

Time constraints are powerful tools. However, don't forget, with great power comes great responsibility (sorry, geek attack!).

Identify a goal-achievement strategy

Setting goals, and figuring out a strategy of how you are going to get there, are not the same thing. Inexperienced triathletes, and even experienced triathletes, often set long-term goals, including outcome goals – 'I'm going to win the big race at the end of the season' – with little or no idea how they are going to achieve them.

For example, your end-of-season goal is to compete in your first half-Ironman distance race. Great! Are practice races going to play a part in your preparation? A half-Ironman distance is a long way without some shorter practice races to help get you physically and mentally prepared for the task. Perhaps you can do a short sprint triathlon race staged by your local triathlon club a month or two into your training, then a couple of increasingly longer, more crowded triathlons as the season progresses. They may only be 'practice' races in your training schedule, but nothing gets the nerves and adrenaline flowing faster than standing on the water's edge with a thousand other competitors ready for the sound of the starter's gun!

You know the phrase 'The best laid plans of mice and men ...' It means that no matter how much planning, there is always the unexpected waiting around the corner to disrupt proceedings.

A good strategy will help you achieve your longer-term goals, but be flexible enough to allow for changes at a moment's notice, perhaps because of injury, and still be able to move forward toward those longer-term goals.

See how they combine to reach the next level of goals

Here's a tenuous analogy. Think of goals as a jigsaw puzzle. The finished jigsaw puzzle is your long-term goal. The hundreds of puzzle pieces are the hundreds of smaller goals you have to piece together over the years to get to your long-term goal. If you want to take the analogy further, then the edge puzzle pieces are your short-term goals. You start with those because they make the puzzle easier to complete.

How you eventually complete the puzzle may not be the same way for everyone. For example, some people like to work their way into the middle from the edges, or focus on the same colour pieces first. However, one thing is for sure: the puzzle pieces all fit together in a complementary way once the puzzle is complete.

That is exactly the same for long-term goals. Two people may well have the same long-term goal, but how they achieve it depends on their individual strategies and their short- and medium-term goals. The one thing that is certain is that those smaller goals will eventually prove to be complementary, combining in a progressive and positive way to culminate in the successful attainment of that long-term goal.

So when setting goals, see the big picture as well as the smaller ones. See how they will all fit together and help you achieve those long-term goals.

When you have several goals, give each a priority

One of the keys to goal setting is not to have too many at once. However, whether you have three or a dozen, you will have to prioritise them in relation both to each other and to your overall long-term goals.

This is because, due to the sheer volume of training required for improvement in triathlon, it does tend to eat into time allocated to other meaningful activities in the life of the triathlete. Prioritising is a must for those that need to time-manage their day, and stay sane while they are doing it.

A number of factors could impact your goals, and even influence what is possible in a given time frame. For example, the training schedule itself. What sort of schedule is possible? There may be times in the year where your 'pay the rent/mortgage/bills' work is busier than at other times. If your work is seasonal and summer is the busiest time, then do not set your major race goal of the season to be an Ironman in September! The amount of time you will have to donate to training for such a major event will eat into your day. And no matter how fit you think you are, Ironman training will leave you tired.

What type of training is available to you? If you are working or living in a limited space, you may not have access to enough quality training opportunities to realistically tackle a half-Ironman as your next race goal. You need access to long swims, bikes and runs. You may not always have access to back-up training opportunities such as a treadmill or a stationary bike trainer. And if one of the disciplines is more of a specialty, such as mountain biking instead of road biking, then you need to have access to off-road trails to practise off-road cycling technique.

Maybe you do not have volume training available and instead just have an hour a day, at most; then your triathlon goals should consider that. Sprint triathlons are far more realistic as a race goal, when only shorter and more focused training sessions are available, and longer-distance triathlons that require more volume in training are not.

Aside from training, scheduling, work and the need to sleep, there needs to be some quality down time, especially if you have a family. The longer the triathlon race planned, the more the training required to successfully complete it with minimum risk of injury. Quality family time should be at the top of the list in the continually evolving 'There are not enough hours in the day' daily/weekly schedule breakdown.

A set time each day should be set aside for family. You do not want to alienate your family, as they will be a major contributing factor to success in triathlon. The same for having a social life. You need down time.

This is a book for masters athletes and older, which means the importance of sleep can never be underestimated. It should be a major priority. You may have been able to burn the candle at both ends when you were 25, but when you're 50 the wick starts to look a little depleted! Sleep is essential to triathlon training recovery and improving performance, as well as attitude.

Priorities are essential when setting out on your triathlon journey. However, every person is different – different in why they do triathlon, the time they have to dedicate to the sport and the goals they want to achieve in it. Setting priorities, though, is one of the keys to success, as is the need to be open and flexible to the ever-changing needs of the sport, and life in general.

Set practice as well as competition goals

While many people associate goal setting with competition, setting practice and training goals are also essential to increased performance. We spend most of our time practising and in training, so it makes sense that practice and training goals can contribute to performance increases.

For example, it may take you 10 minutes to run 100 yards in a wetsuit (from the end of the swimming stage), take off the wetsuit, put on your bike gear and start on the bike leg. With practice, you could very feasibly reduce that by two or three minutes. Those minutes can make a big difference at the end of the run leg. Practising transitions is an often overlooked part of training, but one which can save you sometimes minutes in race time, with no energy expended at all.

Practising with good technique is essential to performance improvement as well. As a result, setting technique improvement goals is vital to improved performance and will also help reduce the risk of injury.

Set positive goals as opposed to negative goals

As stated in the previous chapter, I believe that once you have reached the level of fitness required to complete the race you want to complete, then triathlon becomes 90 per cent mental. It becomes a fundamentally mental sport, in

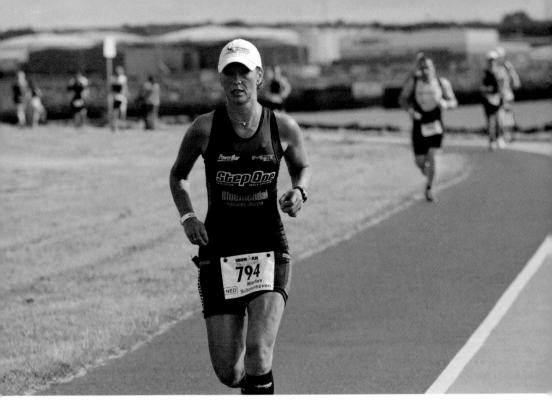

both training and competing. Wherever possible the mental emphasis should have a positive spin. That also applies to goals and goal setting.

How does that work? Instead of setting a goal such as 'I need to stop running flat-footed', which is negative, the goal should be phrased, and the subsequent focus should be placed upon, 'I need to focus every step on striking the ground first with my heel and then rolling it forward and pushing off with the ball of my foot and my toes', which is positive.

For the swim, instead of 'I need to stop keeping my arms straight in my stroke pull-through', it should be 'I need to focus on maintaining a high elbow and keeping my pull-through hand closer to my chest on every stroke'.

Wherever possible, a culture of positivity needs to be established in both training and racing.

Be flexible

Flexibility, in both training and during a race, is an essential ingredient to triathlon success. Having goals and a strategy to accomplish them is essential, but flexibility is vital.

Circumstances in training can change in an instant – even mid-session – just as conditions during a race can change on a single stride or stroke pull-through. Injuries are a very real and constant threat. A slight twinge in the first 10 minutes of a training session, for example, may mean you need to ease off and reduce the intensity, or to stop altogether to make sure more damage is not being done by continuing.

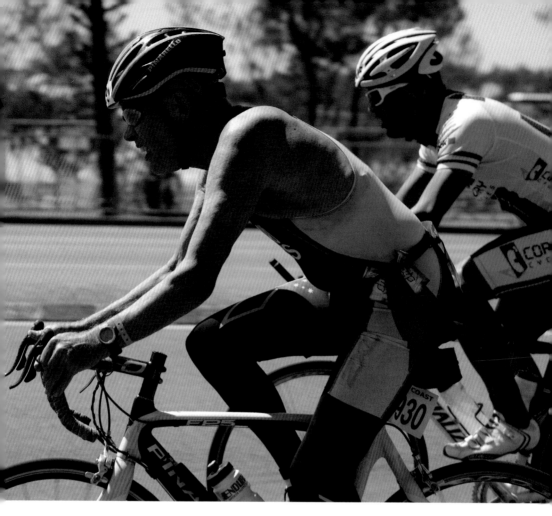

More than that, though, your circumstances, training environment or conditions can also change overnight. You may have a long run set up for Saturday, but on Friday you may have to get on a plane. If you can't move the run to Sunday, or it conflicts with another essential element of your training, or your life, you may have to just miss out on that run that week. It is not the end of the world.

Being inflexible and stressing over changes in your schedule or training – maybe even a small but essential change in technique – impacts the positive outlook that is essential to successful triathlon.

Mechanical problems happen on a regular basis if you put in a lot of bike training. Be prepared for them with good maintenance on your equipment, but also with a positive attitude that is ready and flexible enough to switch the session to something else should the situation demand it.

Be vested in setting goals

One of the great motivating tools for any coach, when setting goals, is to have the athlete contribute to the task. As a triathlete, you should be vested in the goals that are set for you. Obviously if you don't have a coach, then you don't have a choice. In that case, you are setting your own goals already. However, if you are thinking of setting goals and targetting performance improvement, you should consider having a personal coach.

Even if you do have a coach, in discussing with them what you want out of triathlon and your season, contribute to the ways that your goals can be achieved. For example, understand why you need to improve your technique and how you can improve it by setting technique goals. That way, when you are tired and under stress during training, it becomes easier to understand what you need to focus on and be more of a motivational tool to complete it correctly.

A word about fun and doing the things you like. Triathlon should be fun. You should enjoy doing it. So make sure you include a healthy dose of the things you like in your training. Obviously, the things you like are more likely to be the things you are good at, because they are the things you do most, because you like them the best. Yes, it is cyclical! Similarly, the things you do badly are the things you probably do least of. However, in addressing your shortfalls, make sure what you enjoy is included. That is not going to happen unless you become vested in the goal-setting process yourself.

In addition, if there are things in training you do not like, find alternatives that address the same problem or coaching focus, but are accomplished in a different way that you like better. That will be even more incentive to reach the goal, because you suggested an alternative to your coach's ideas, so you have to ensure it will succeed!

Set complementary team or training partner goals

Triathlon is an individual sport. There is no one else out there to help you when the chips are down and you are cramping with six miles to go in the half-marathon leg of your half-Ironman. That said, having a training partner, or training with a group, can be very motivational.

Ideally, your training partner or group should have roughly the same athletic abilities. It may not stay that way, but initially they will. So establishing a collective goal or two can be hugely beneficial and motivating. Even better, if your training partner is signed up for the same race as you, then that is only going to help.

A training partner helps motivate on a day-to-day basis. Remember, though, that because triathlon has three different disciplines, you do not have to have the same training partner for all of them. Having a training partner with the same running ability, for example, can lead to mutually beneficial running goals, even if that person is not your training partner in the other disciplines. Any time their training goals match yours, you have a built-in motivational tool.

Collective pain is easier to endure than individual pain!

Personality and individual differences

Individual personality plays an important role in any goal setting. It is not just about setting goals. Goals have to be realistic in terms of both the physical demands and the personality of the individual involved.

For example, if you are not a morning person, don't schedule workouts at the crack of dawn before you go to work. If you do, you are going to find it increasingly difficult to get motivated that early in the morning and you are not going to have much fun doing the scheduled sessions.

When setting goals it is also vital to be honest with yourself about how ambitious you are. If you are a 'high achiever', you should have no problem accepting difficult (but realistic) goals to pursue. But if you harbour more modest ambitions, or may be low on self-confidence, it is important to accept that and gravitate towards more realistic goals. In either case the aim should be to strike a balance between aiming high and avoiding biting off more than you can chew, and each triathlete will have to determine how to strike that balance for themselves.

Seek support of goals

Support plays a major role in reaching goals. Triathlons, especially the longer distances, involve such a major commitment to training that there is less chance of success without the support of family and friends, for example. If you have a family, their close support can be the difference between success and failure.

Additionally, the most successful goal achievers are those that seek feedback for their efforts, most often from a coach. However, for anyone that does not have a coach, feedback is just as essential. So a form of feedback that should be utilised is keeping a concise training log and being as objective as you can with your ongoing evaluation of training progress.

MOTIVATION

Motivation and goals are entwined. An understanding of what motivates a person will help in the design of a realistic set of personalised goals. Focusing on those goals will motivate because the two are connected.

That said, the easiest way to get motivated is to love what you are doing and, ultimately, to have fun doing it. Of course, you are unlikely to be having much fun in the middle of a high-intensity workout where muscles are screaming out for you to stop and your lungs can't find enough oxygen. Overall, though, you need to be enjoying what you are doing.

However, if, after so many months of triathlon training, you are not enjoying it, or you are not having any fun, you should ask yourself 'Why am I doing this?' It is the same question you should have asked yourself when you embarked on your initial triathlon training programme, and you should ask every year before the season begins. If you increasingly view upcoming training sessions with dread and apprehension, those months of training may give you a more enlightened appreciation for what makes you tick, and you should be able to identify what you need to change to make training more enjoyable.

SMART GOALS

A quick and easy way to ensure you are setting useful goals is to use the often-quoted SMART acronym. SMART goals are those that are:

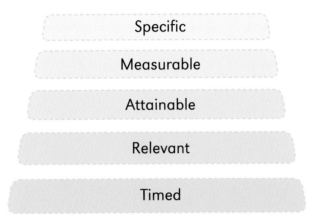

Specific

Measurable

Attainable

Relevant

Timed

These criteria are all discussed in this chapter. Make sure they are met!

CONCLUSION

It is plain and simple: setting goals works, whether in triathlon or life in general. Goals are a way of motivating and a way to provide direction. However, they have to be realistic and achievable.

One of the big problems for goal setting in masters athletes is that they tend to base their goals on a fitness level from 20 years before. As described elsewhere in this book, fitness, endurance, muscle mass, bone density, power and strength all decline with age. However, how much they decline depends on training, how much high-intensity work is done, and the level of fitness to begin with.

As a result, it is even more important for masters athletes to be realistic in the goals they set and to understand what is motivating them to participate in triathlons in the first place.

06

PLANNNG AND PREPARATION

THREE MASTERS CONSIDERATIONS DISCUSSED IN THIS CHAPTER:

- Planning and preparation is even more important for masters athletes than younger triathletes. As the body ages, its ability to think and react on the fly diminishes. But given enough planning and preparation time it can still perform at a high level.

- Effective time management skills are not a luxury for masters athletes – they are essential. Available time will always be at a premium for 'type A' triathletes, whatever the age, but the ability of the body and mind to maintain continuous day-long frantic pace will decline.

- For most masters triathletes, the memory is not what it was! So more often than not, well-thought-out checklists will save the day and reduce stress.

Success in triathlon is defined by preparation. The better the preparation and more effective the planning, the more likely you are to succeed. Triathlon is all about planning and being prepared. And then it is all about being flexible enough to change those plans as conditions, and often injuries, dictate.

The harder and more complex the training, and the greater the commitment to the sport for the triathlete, the more important it is to have plans and to be prepared – for everything from weekly training schedules to season race calendars around which training revolves.

WHY PLAN?

Planning and preparation help achieve goals. Well-thought-out planning allows you to achieve your step-by-step short-term goals, which in turn allows you to reach the important medium and longer term goals. Planning lets a triathlete define a strategy to achieve those goals and determine a time frame for completion.

With triathlon, if something bad can happen, it probably will. Planning allows us to prepare for the worst-case scenario, and then work backwards from there.

Triathlon is all about flexibility and being able to adapt to unfolding events – mechanicals, injuries, even challenging weather. Planning for those worst-case scenarios, and being fully prepared by practising repairs or acclimatising to adverse weather conditions such as heat, increases the likelihood of success.

Importantly, good planning allows for the removal of the duplication of effort. Triathlon is time-consuming enough without doing unnecessary work and training. This applies to general triathlon administration as well as training schedules and workouts. Any time you can remove extra, unnecessary work, no matter how small the time and effort saving, consider it a success.

In the short term, that could be as simple as a single trip to the bike shop as a result of writing a comprehensive list of everything you will need for the next two weeks, instead of just stopping by twice a week to pick up supplies as training and travel demands. Alternatively, it could be registering early for a race, or scheduling picking up your race packet and attending the mandatory race meeting at the same time, in order to avoid separate trips to the race venue the day before the event when you have to also drop off your bike.

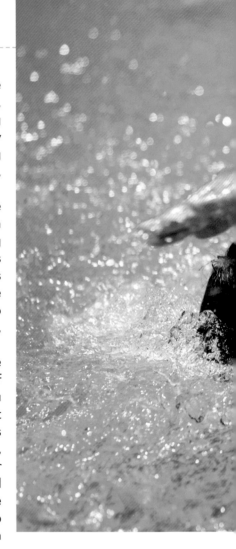

Last, but certainly not least, planning allows you to realistically evaluate the cost of triathlon, and what you can reasonably expect to accomplish based on your economic circumstances. Do not register for an exotic Ironman halfway around the world if you have no money to spare from one payday to the next! Be realistic in what you can accomplish.

Aside from the cost of entry into a race – for example, a half-Ironman is typically around £150 ($250), while a full Ironman is £300–400 ($500–600) – if you are travelling to the race, costs can mount up quickly. If the race is overseas, costs can get extremely high.

For example, take bike travel cases. Not only do you have to contend with the high cost of airline tickets, or more accurately the exorbitant extra fees for airline fuel, but every airline charges extra for bike travel cases. Some airlines charge as much as £130 ($200) each way for a bike travel case if you are flying internationally. Also, if you plan on a taxi from the destination airport to

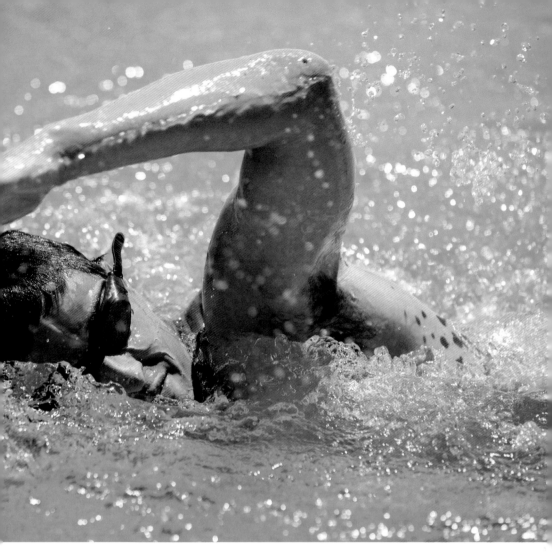

your hotel, expect to pay extra for taking the bike case with you in the vehicle. Most of the time a minivan-style taxi will be required.

I used a minibus taxi at one overseas race to get from the airport to my hotel and the taxi driver charged a flat fee per person in the large passenger van, which was fair enough. But then I was charged an extra charge the equivalent of another person just for the bike case, even though the case was in the storage section of the van at the back and not taking up any seats! But what can you do in that situation? A bike case will not fit into a typical taxi, so you have to use a larger-than-normal vehicle. The result was another £15 ($25) each way for the bike case, from the airport to the hotel and back. It all adds up, especially overseas. Maybe advanced planning and research can eliminate the unforeseen and get additional discounts.

In general, check the travel bike case charges before you book your airline tickets and expect to also add as much as £30 ($50) extra for taxi charges from the airport to where you are staying. As a result, be sure to ask yourself if it would be more cost-effective, and certainly less hassle, to just ship your triathlon bike, depending on the race.

TIME MANAGEMENT

Preparation and time management go hand in hand. If you have bad time management, the chance of being fully prepared for a race decreases. Triathlon training is time-consuming and there are only so many hours in a day. For most people with other commitments – such as family, work and a social life – having, or acquiring, effective time management skills are a fundamental part of their triathlon lifestyle.

If someone cannot get all their workouts in, then there is a good chance they are lacking in their planning and preparation. If that is not the case, then they need to take a hard look at their prioritisation skills.

You may love a specific pool for swim training workouts. However, if it takes an hour round trip just to get to that pool, it may be better to go to your closest pool instead and use that extra hour for something more important than driving in a car to a workout.

Time management skills allow you to effectively plan and prepare your triathlon schedule and strategy. This can be a major problem for older athletes, however, especially if they have not had to keep a tight rein on their daily hours throughout their life. You *can* teach an old dog new tricks, but it takes hard work to change a mind that is set in its laid-back ways.

However, there is a parallel between time management skills and triathlon. Staying focused is essential to time management discipline. In addition, staying focused and not letting yourself get distracted by things that don't matter is also vital to triathlon, both in training and racing.

ORGANISATIONAL SKILLS

Organisational skills are another invaluable tool in any triathlete's arsenal. If your organisational skills are lacking, it is time to take a class or get some personal tuition in how to organise effectively.

Aside from the planning and preparation of your training schedule and goal achievement strategies, organisation is at the very heart of a stress-free triathlon lifestyle. It is a priceless tool used in every facet from preparing for a long ride, or a trip to the gym, to how to slide through transitions with the minimum of fuss and wasted time on race day.

Organising is deceptively step-by-step – begin at the beginning and end at the end. In these modern days of 'I want it now', it is almost counter-intuitive to demand time to slow down, while you meticulously make sure everything has been accounted for before moving on to the next step. The end comes once you have made sure everything in each step on the way has been completed effectively.

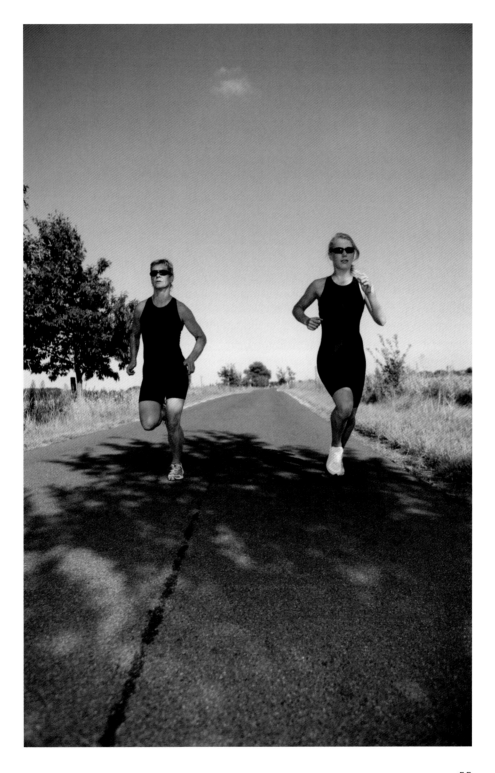

CHECKLISTS

You cannot beat a good checklist! And why would you want to? Why would you leave something to chance when every item could instead be written down in front of you, in the order they have to be completed?

Checklists can be indispensable. Checklists can be used for everything from grocery shopping for a healthy diet, to what is required in transitioning from the bike to the run in a race, to pre-race registration to-do requirements, to pre-training equipment preparation.

Checklists are a great organisational tool. They focus thoughts and allow a triathlete to pre-visualise their actions at the same time.

Checklists can also be used in remembering correct technique. Simply write down the main points of a technique, in the order they are to be accomplished, and put that checklist in a place where you can see it – before, during and after your workout. Checklists can be an aid to mental preparation as well as physical application of techniques and goals.

MENTAL PREPARATION

As will be repeated many times in this book, once you have achieved a certain level of fitness and technique, triathlon becomes predominantly a mental sport.

Training the mind is as important as training the body. Mental preparation is as important as physical preparation. Physical fitness becomes useless if your mind is unprepared for the task and inevitable punishment and pain that lie ahead. The mind must be prepared for anything that crosses its path – in training, during the race, and in life generally.

Just as there is a need to prepare the body to cope with the physical demands of such a tough sport as triathlon, so there is a need to prepare the mind for the mental demands that are going to come.

KEEP A FITNESS BAG WITH YOU IN THE CAR

Triathlon, and especially triathlon training, is all about flexibility, and the need to change plans and take advantage of opportunities at a moment's notice. So it is a good idea to keep a small back-up fitness bag with you in your car at all times. You never know when training plans will have to be changed because of work or other commitments, making it impossible to adhere to the pre-planned schedule for the week. Also, there are times when the opportunity to snatch an hour of unexpected training will arise, to supplement the regular training schedule's change of plan.

There is no need to keep much in the back-up bag – just basic run, swim and gym gear. In its barest form, that would be:

- a pair of running shoes;
- running socks;

- a good pair of triathlon shorts that can be used for running, swimming and gym workouts;
- a proper running top made of breathable, wicking material;
- a pair of swim goggles;
- a towel;
- a water bottle.

Be prepared for the unexpected, and do not use the unexpected as a reason not to adhere to your triathlon training plan, unless there really is no other way.

PRE-PLAN ALTERNATIVE BIKE AND RUN TRAINING ROUTES

In keeping with the spirit of the back-up bag described above, keep a list of alternative riding and running routes available that can be used to replace any intended training routes. If you are unfamiliar with them, print out maps and directions for the routes and file them beforehand in a small database of alternative routes. Then, for whatever reason, if you need to change a planned training route, a printed map is already to hand without the need to access additional links in the technology/Internet chain.

If you are travelling and intend to train while away, make sure you have a list of alternative cycling or running routes wherever you will be staying. Print out maps as necessary beforehand in case access to the Internet or printer are unavailable. Take away as many reasons to say 'not today' as you can by effective pre-planning.

CONCLUSION

The bottom line is that the more prepared you are, the more likely you are to succeed. Effective planning helps remove stress and the likelihood that unexpected elements will derail a well-thought-out training and race schedule. The more planning and preparation, the more control we have over our own destiny, and the less can go wrong.

In addition, the older the triathlete, the less they should rely on memory or unplanned and unprepared-for fly-by-the-seat-of-your-pants decision making!

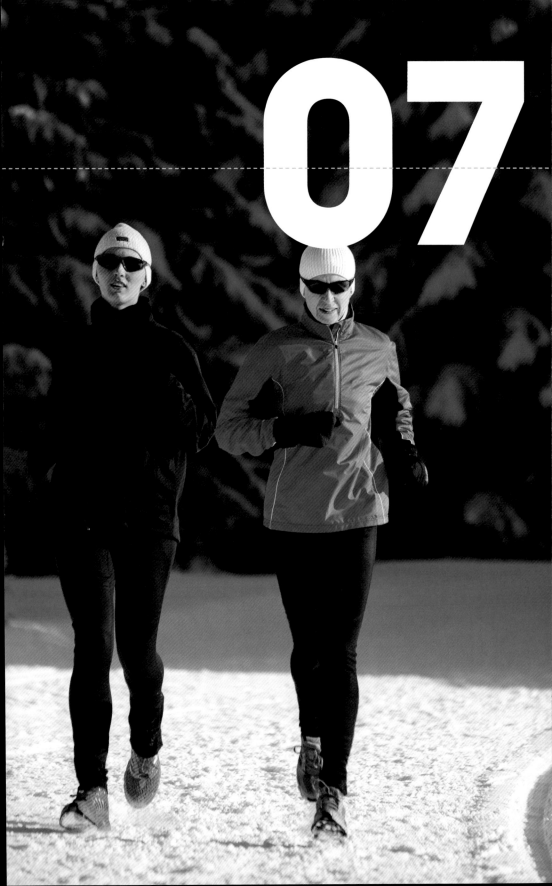

07

TRAINING PROGRAMMES

Improved performance in triathlon is all about incremental gains, which come from well-thought-out training programmes and workout schedules. Training programmes or plans need to be tailored to the individual triathlete – their strengths and weaknesses, their likes and dislikes, their physical fitness and their tendency to get injured. For masters triathletes, one size definitely does not fit all, and generic training schedules, especially for masters triathletes, are not a good idea.

This chapter does not offer sample training plans. Instead, it covers what a triathlete, and especially a masters triathlete, should be considering as they try to figure out a training programme in their move from beginner to intermediate levels.

As the start of each year swings around, all triathletes, from beginner to pro, have to determine what they want from the upcoming season. For the most part, the questions raised in this chapter should be asked by every triathlete at every level every year. It is never a bad thing to re-evaluate your reasons for doing triathlon, as they may have changed or evolved without you realising.

The first issue for any triathlete to consider, then, is what training schedule to commit to over the coming season. An advanced triathlon programme will include endurance training, low- and high-intensity workout sessions, technique and technical instruction, stretching, weight training, discipline-specific strength training, and, last but by no means least, a good diet with enough nutrition and calories to allow your body to function at its optimum level.

THE TRIATHLON YEAR

First things first, though. What needs to be considered when deciding upon a training programme?

To reflect on that, we need to break down the triathlon year into its simplest form. Triathlon training is essentially year-round. However, it does have its race season, mostly during the spring, summer and autumn, and its off-season, usually in the winter months. That is not always true, of course, because triathlon races are available all over the world.

The off-season, which lasts 3–4 months, is usually the time when a triathlete puts in long hours of steady training at mostly lower intensities, building up an endurance base that they will build upon in the run-up to race season.

A typical race season is split up around two or three targeted main races. These are the 'A' races around which training revolves. This dividing of the season is often called periodisation, or sometimes segmentation, and entails organising training into progressive periods or blocks of time. Each period consists of 2–3 months or so, depending on how many 'A' races are included in a season, and culminates in one of the 'A' races.

Triathletes often do additional races, perhaps local running races or sprint triathlons, but those races are usually considered more 'training races', entered to build speed or get familiar with the chaos of race day when the result doesn't mean a great deal and the pressure is off.

Whatever the length of each segment between 'A' races, the training weeks are typically divided into different blocks. The sequence of blocks usually start with a short recovery of a week or two from the previous race, then a base endurance phase, then an adaptation phase, then a race-specific phase for whatever race is next coming up, and then a taper, which helps the triathlete peak for that next race.

However, having established the basic structure of the triathlon year, which type of training schedule or plan is decided upon, along with the resulting training schedule, depends on a number of questions.

MICROCYCLES, MESOCYCLES AND MACROCYCLES

A quick word is necessary on the often-seen coaching terms *microcycle*, *mesocycle* and *macrocycle*, most often used in endurance and progressive resistance types of training. In short, these terms correspond to a short-term cycle of training, a medium-term cycle, and a long-term cycle. The actual length of the cycles depends on the coach. Often, though, a microcyle consists of a seven-day block of training. A mesocycle can be anything from 2–3 weeks or a 4-week block to several months. The term macrocycle mostly refers to an overall training time frame, perhaps a season or a calendar year.

QUESTIONS TO CONSIDER

While this book is intended for those triathletes who have at least a rudimentary knowledge of swimming, biking and running, it is always a good idea to revisit basic technique, even for the pros. All triathletes can benefit from increased technical excellence.

At the start of each season, the following questions should be asked of yourself, even though you asked them last season, and the season before that. So before considering a choice of training programme, consider these basic questions, because it is only by answering them honestly that you can know what it is you want from your commitment to triathlon.

What are your triathlon goals and your life goals?

Hopefully, those two questions have complementary answers; if not, then 'Houston, we have a problem!' Triathlon goals should not dominate every other aspect of your life. In fact, triathlon goals should complement your life goals and should work in unison to create a better life and lifestyle.

If triathlon goals dominate every aspect of your life, you should stop and ask why. Is it you who is letting them dominate, whether consciously or sub-consciously? If it is, again, you need to find out why.

Why are you doing triathlon and what level do you want to participate in?

Why are you doing triathlon? This question will keep repeating itself each year, and every time you are having a tough time in training or in a race. Just like a patient's initial answers on the therapist's couch, most initial answers are superficial and it is only by digging deeper that the true reasons comes out.

Also, there will be a question as to what level of the sport do you want to reach and how hard do you want to train. Many 'type A' triathletes gravitate towards high-intensity, 'bring on the pain' workouts and training schedules. As a result, the subsequent danger becomes overtraining and burnout. Alternatively, many also like the lower intensity, and long hours, that training for an Ironman or half-Ironman distance race demands.

Obviously, if you prefer the longer, lower-intensity training, forcing too many high-intensity workouts on your body every week may eventually lead to burnout, and certainly a lack of motivation when it comes to getting up and through the door to the next training session. However, one or two high-intensity workouts are necessary every week, especially for masters athletes, as I emphasise throughout this book.

So a simple question such as 'Why are you doing triathlon?' should not be answered superficially. It needs some serious thought. The answer will form the basic foundation of an athlete's triathlon training.

How much time do you have to train?

This is a question that requires a brutally honest answer! For most people, a serious commitment to triathlon training and racing, and the triathlon lifestyle that goes along with it, means they will have to give something else up that is already established in their lives. Triathlon training is a time-consuming business.

At its most basic level of training, the beginner's time commitment will be at least 5–6 hours a week. Even at that level, it is only 45–60 minutes for 4 days during the week, and then a longer ride of 90–120 minutes one day at the weekend. That hardly qualifies as a serious commitment. Many would view that number of hours as the absolute minimum required to train for three disciplines. A more realistic figure for anyone wishing to move up a level would be 6–8 hours a week. That would equate to at least four 1-hour sessions during the week and a 2-hour ride at the weekend.

As a rule of thumb, 6–8 hours of training a week will work if you are targeting a sprint, or maybe an Olympic distance triathlon race. Anything longer, such as a half-Ironman distance race, will require more hours than that.

Why? Because if your bike leg in the race (half-Ironman) is going to take you 3½ hours, then your long ride every week in training cannot be 2 hours.

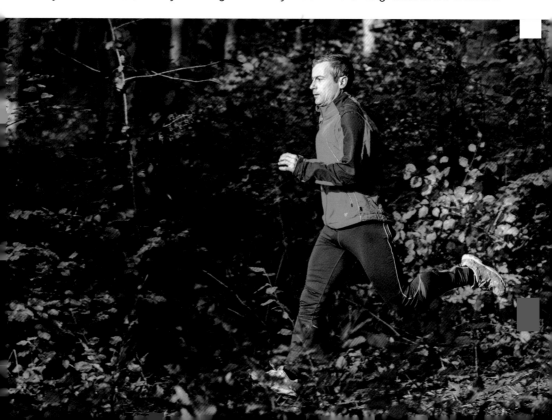

That is not the way triathlon training works. And even then, a half-marathon to finish will take close to another 2½ hours, so your long training run each week cannot be 1 hour.

Time is a hurdle every triathlete has to overcome. It comes back to challenge you on multiple fronts and in multiple forms throughout your triathlon life.

You may want to aim for a half-Ironman distance race by the end of this year, but the reality may be that you only have regular training time available every week to target a sprint triathlon instead.

Do you have an endurance base already and how long before your first race?

To state the obvious, you can get away with less endurance base if you are planning a sprint triathlon than if you are planning a half-Ironman distance race. If you have some sort of endurance base, even a little, it will change the initial approach to the early part of your training programme.

Having any sort of endurance base will also affect how quickly an athlete can participate in their first race. The one thing you do not want to do is race too quickly, before your body is ready.

A triathlete needs to have had at least some progressive training structure before that first race, culminating in a well-executed taper leading up to race day.

If you do not have an endurance base in all three disciplines, there is no quick fix to getting it. You have to put in the training hours. That means bumping back your first race until you know your body can cope with the higher intensity of racing a triathlon.

Do you have any prior injuries that could pose a problem?

The first step that needs to be taken before committing to a lifetime of pain and pleasure with the triathlon lifestyle is to make sure you are physically capable of completing the ongoing weekly hours of training without damaging your body. So go and see a doctor. This is especially true for masters athletes, and doubly true for those over 50 years of age. The physical decline of a body accelerates after the age of 50, and depends on the fitness of the athlete.

If you have the time, and the financial resources, you should also get such things as your running gait analysed. For those coming from a running background, any major problem with running gait would probably have become apparent over the years of run training, but not necessarily.

Injuries are like a leaking roof. The leak in the roof is rarely where the water comes into the room below. It leaks in through one part of the roof and then travels along the eaves before dropping down and seeping through the ceiling on the other side of the house. Hamstring problems, for example, could have dozens of causes, many of them linked to stresses and strains placed on muscles far away from the hamstrings.

Similarly, a bad neck could easily be caused by lower back problems, which could be caused by weak muscles on one side of a leg, leading to an unduly lopsided running gait.

Previous injuries can develop into a future problem if they go unaddressed. There is always a reason for an injury, and much of the time that reason is not the result of a violent impact or accident. Most injuries to triathletes are related to training, overuse or the result of bad technique.

A recurring injury may prevent you from doing the long hours of training required to compete safely at an Ironman distance, or any of the longer distances. That same recurring injury may not, however, prevent you from competing in short and sprint triathlons.

The important thing is to acknowledge previous injuries, find out the reason they occurred, and take those findings into account when planning the upcoming triathlon training and racing season.

Are you overweight?

For many, this is a tough question to answer. Many people are in denial about their own weight. That said, however, the desire to lose weight is one of the most common reasons to take up triathlon or move on from the beginner's level.

When planning a training programme, and a more detailed weekly workout schedule, being overweight can be a major initial factor. This is especially true for those without a long history of endurance training, or who do not have much experience in regular, managed physical exercise.

The danger is especially relevant for those who are severely overweight. These people should avoid running completely until they have lost some of the weight, and instead concentrate on the two disciplines that do not place so much strain on the knees – swimming and biking. The strain on the knees, even for those who are not overweight, is considerable. For those carrying extra weight the danger of future long-term injury as a result of running training is considerable.

With swimming, the entire weight of the body is supported by water. As most of the work in swimming for a triathlete is in the upper body – because you are saving the lower body muscles for the bike and the run – the danger then becomes overuse or extra strain placed on the arms and shoulders by the extra bodyweight. However, swimming carries the least risk in training for someone who is overweight, providing you are applying correct technique and are under competent coaching supervision.

With biking, a severely overweight person should focus training on a stationary bicycle at home or in the gym, to take advantage of the increased stability, controlled effort and terrain demands, and to reduce the risk of on-road accidents. Once they have lost some weight they can move to limited cycling on flat roads, because hills will place extra stress on knees and muscles.

The main rule for overweight athletes, then, is to avoid running at the start of any training programme. Concentrate instead on developing a healthy, nutritious diet that encourages weight loss, and begin working out only with swimming and a stationary biking. Once a given target weight loss has been reached, some moderate running can be introduced to the training programme.

What should you focus on?

You need to have a plan, Stan, and you need to figure it out early. You need a focus for your upcoming year of triathlon training and racing. The difficult part of that, though, is that the answer on what to focus on can prove elusive, at least initially. 'Getting better at triathlon' is too vague an answer . It needs to be more specific. Without that answer though, you cannot really decide on a training programme for the upcoming season. See Chapter 5 (pages 36–49) for more on goal setting.

Of course, you can change the plan midway through the season, and being flexible is part of the key to success in triathlon. However, one of the harsh realities of triathlon is that the entry list for races, especially Ironman and half-Ironman distances, fill up many months in advance, if not a year before the event.

So changing your focus mid-season (unless you have an injury, of course) may be a challenge, because you may not get the races you want, or you may have to travel farther afield to get one. It is a problem that could have been averted if more time had been spent on finding the answers to questions at the beginning of the triathlon year.

CONCLUSION

A triathlete's season-long training programme gets to the very heart and soul of why they want to train and compete in triathlon. To get the most out of training and racing though, a triathlete must fully comprehend why they are doing it in the first place, what they want to achieve by doing it, and the goals they hope to accomplish. That realisation has to come as a result of the questions asked at the very start of the triathlon journey.

Because of that – and especially for masters athletes, who must contend with both the natural aging process of the human body and their own individual physical traits, strengths, weaknesses and injury histories – a generic, off-the-shelf training schedule will not work. A training schedule for a masters triathlete needs to be custom-tailored for each person if they hope to avoid injury and optimise triathlon performance gains.

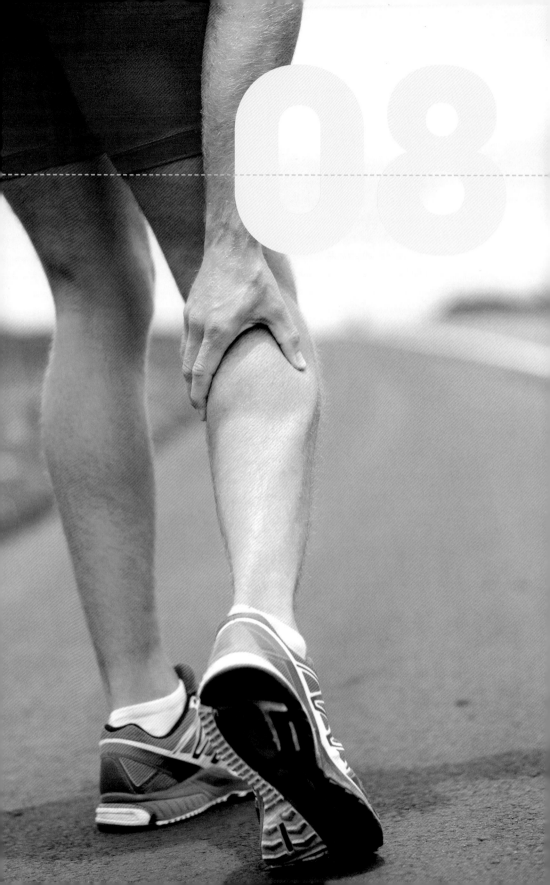

08

MUSCLES AND INJURY PREVENTION

THREE MASTERS CONSIDERATIONS DISCUSSED IN THIS CHAPTER:

- Masters athletes are more prone to injury, so train with injury prevention in mind.

- The older an athlete, the more stresses and strains are placed on the body, so maintaining correct technique is a vital weapon in preventing injury.

- Strength and power are two casualties of age. Strength training is essential to older athletes in helping to main correct technique as fatigue sets in, and in compensating for the loss of muscle mass.

One of the most obvious differences in training between the ages is the increased danger of injury in older athletes – loss of muscle and bone mass, declining VO$_2$ max, loss of elasticity and flexibility in muscles, tendons and ligaments, along with an increase in the possibility of overuse and damage from general wear and tear. That said, knowing the increased danger, any masters triathlete would do well to adopt a more proactive approach to injury prevention to stay fit and on track with their training.

However, this is triathlon. With the amount of hours needed to train for three disciplines, and the extra stresses that are placed on the body as a result, it is inevitable that, without careful attention, at some point the body is going to break down.

The key, then, is to try and prevent that happening. One of the main weapons against injury is to train 'defensively.' In other words, train with one eye on performance improvement and the other eye on injury prevention.

As mentioned, injury prevention is even more important as the body ages, as the flexibility and elasticity in the joints, muscles, tendons and ligaments declines, and recovery from both training and racing takes a little longer. So plan your training, and your schedule, with injury avoidance in the back of your mind.

While you can never be sure where and how an injury is going to strike, there are a number of fundamental defensive tips that can be taken into account as you ramp up the intensity and focus in training.

PREVENTING INJURY
Custom exercises and workout schedules

The older an athlete gets, the more a 'one-size-fits-all' generic approach to training schedules and workouts does not work. Custom training programmes are essential for masters athletes hoping to maximise performance improvements and minimise injury. How we age differs from person to person. Even two triathletes of the same age, gender, ability and current social environment will be different in how they cope and adapt to the same training schedule.

Muscle mass decline, loss of bone density, VO_2 max decline, strength and power declines all differ between athletes and with age. One of the most essential tools in the fight against injury in masters athletes is the ability for their coach to adapt their ongoing workout schedule according to injury, fatigue, motivational, overuse and physiological factors.

Warm-up and cool-down

It is essential to injury prevention that you warm up before every training session or workout. A regular warm-up should consist of, for example, a ten-minute jog, stretches, and perhaps some muscle-specific drills, such as high knee lift, depending on what the training session emphasis is to be.

There are multiple benefits of an effective warm-up – such as getting the blood circulating through active tissues, obtaining a workable heart rate for exercise, and reducing muscle stiffness.

Do not ignore a proper cool-down after a workout session. It should include stretching and easy movement of the legs, such as an easy bike spin.

Stretching

The cases for and against stretching, and when to do it, ebb and flow like the ocean tides! One thing is for sure, though: stretching is not just for old people. It is for everyone, but perhaps especially for older athletes. Stretching should occur before and after a workout, and during if necessary. Never be afraid to stop at a convenient place in your workout to stretch. Stretching helps maintain a maximum range of motion. That is extremely important as you begin to place unusual stresses and strains on your muscles and joints.

However, the prevailing thought is not to stretch cold muscles. So do not stretch until you have done at least the initial part of your warm-up. An often quoted rule of thumb is not to start serious stretching until you have broken some sort of a sweat.

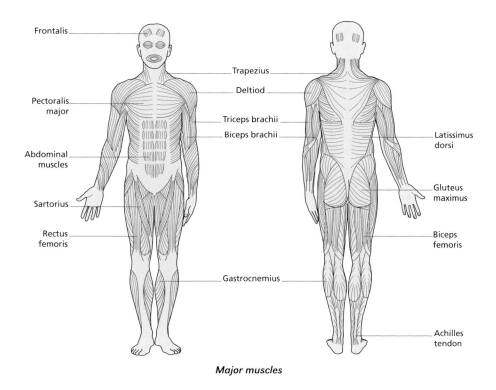

Frontalis

Trapezius

Deltiod

Pectoralis major

Triceps brachii

Biceps brachii

Latissimus dorsi

Abdominal muscles

Sartorius

Gluteus maximus

Rectus femoris

Biceps femoris

Gastrocnemius

Achilles tendon

Major muscles

If something begins to get a little tight during the training session or workout, stop at an appropriate place and stretch. If you feel something getting more than a little tight, stop immediately and stretch. Try and loosen up the tightness. If, after trying to loosen it with stretching and other activities, it still has not loosened, stop the session. Then try and loosen it up outside of training, perhaps with a hot bath or a massage, followed by more stretching.

Every training session and workout should end with stretching as part of your cool-down. Focus on stretching the muscles and the muscle groups that were used the most.

Flexibility

The older someone gets, the more important it is for the body to remain flexible. That applies to muscles and joints, as well as the mind. It is common knowledge that one of the main causes of inactivity in older people is a lack of flexibility in the joints and muscles, which begin to make exercising and staying active harder as the years progress.

Staying active and exercising does not stop the aging process, but there is extensive research to show that it does slow it down considerably. Keeping the muscles and joints flexible is a guaranteed way of helping that slowdown and prevent injuries.

Yoga for example, is an excellent low-impact way to maintain flexibility as you age. It may not directly impact your triathlon personal best times, but it will help your body train consistently by reducing the risk of injury caused by lack of muscle and joint flexibility.

Correct technique

Technique does not need to be perfect, but it needs to be correct. Correct technique means more efficiency, which means less energy used, which means faster times with less effort. Correct technique also reduces the risk of injury.

Even if you choose not to have a 'full-time' coach to oversee your training and write your training schedules, you certainly need a knowledgeable coach, or coaches, that can teach you correct technique for cycling and running, and especially swimming. Of all the disciplines, swimming is the one that benefits most from good technique. Conversely, running is probably the most likely to result in an injury from bad technique.

Gym workouts and strength training

Prolonged correct technique depends on body and muscle strength. As a triathlon race progresses and you become tired, strong muscles help you maintain form, which makes you more efficient, which in turn allows you to use less energy. It also helps prevent a deterioration of form, which will result in unnecessary strains and stresses being placed on the muscles and joints.

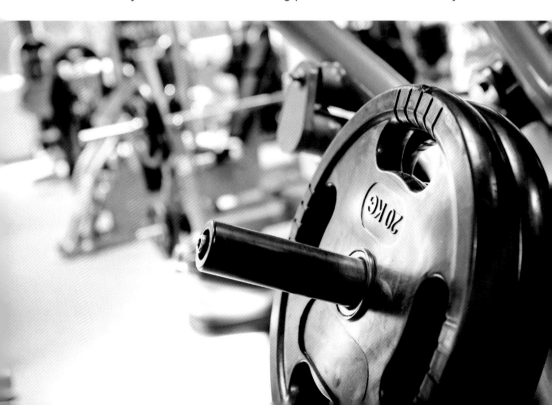

Continued strength workouts throughout the year help strong technique, even for those who have muscle strength. Establishing a discipline-specific training schedule in the gym, targeting muscle groups vital to triathlon techniques, will strengthen muscles.

For example, the common injuries in swimming are to do with the shoulders. The triathlete must learn to recognise the difference between regular workout tiredness and significant aches that could lead to tendonitis. Poor swim technique is one cause of shoulder pain. However, another major reason is weak shoulder muscles or muscles that are underdeveloped. A progressive strength programme designed to strengthen the shoulder muscles will help prevent injury over time.

One of the most significant effects of aging is the loss of muscle mass, especially after the age of 50. Strength training helps combat the deterioration of muscle mass.

Balance

Strength training and the maintenance of muscle mass also contributes in no small part to the ability to maintain balance, especially on uneven ground. Deteriorating balance, and falling as a result, is one of the main causes of injuries in the general aging population.

In addition to weight and strength training aimed at maintaining the necessary muscles for balance, general gym and balance-focused exercises should be included in every masters training schedule on a regular basis. All three disciplines in triathlon require balance, even swimming, and lack of adequate balance in cycling can result in serious injury with the speeds that can be obtained on the bike.

MORE IS NOT ALWAYS BETTER

The phrase 'more is not always better' applies to both volume and intensity, where going longer and harder does not always make you faster and stronger; it can also get you injured. As I have already noted, triathletes typically have 'type A' personalities, where pushing themselves to the limit to succeed is the norm.

However, sometimes that eagerness to push harder and longer needs to be tempered. Triathlon training is also about discipline and incremental performance gains. Many times those gains cannot be achieved by simply going harder and longer.

LISTEN TO YOUR BODY

This is one of the primary rules of injury-free triathlon training. As a triathlete, it is necessary to learn the differences between the aches and soreness of day-to-day hard training, and the dangers of muscle tweaks and pains that could be the indication of a potential injury.

If the usual holdover aches and soreness that most feel at the start of the next day's training session do not subside after the warm-up, or even an extended warm-up, and carry into the actual session for more than a few minutes, care should be taken and a fuller examination of the offending area needs to be made.

If you get a muscle tweak or a pain while training, the best course of action is to slow down, evaluate the situation, and even stop if you need to. It is okay to slow down, even in a race, if you think there could be cause for alarm. However, as mentioned, you have to learn to distinguish between regular training pain and injury pain.

RECOVERY

Scheduled recovery time

Scheduling in recovery time during the week is essential and designed to help your body recover from the demands of training. After your muscles get broken down in training, they require sufficient time to rebuild and come back stronger. Without the time to rebuild, your body will become weaker and weaker, increasing the chance of injury as your muscles become unable to handle the extensive demands of triathlon training.

Sleep

Sleep is the prime time your body has to recover from training. Making sure you have enough sleep each day is as important as your workouts and training schedule. This is especially important for masters athletes. The older one gets, the more important enough sleep becomes.

After a particularly hard training day, you should add extra sleep that night. You should also add extra sleep following a race, especially for longer races (over 2 hours). With the half-Ironman distance, and particularly the full Ironman, you should get as much sleep as you can. No alarm clock for a few days, if that is possible in your life schedule! Give your body the chance to do what it does best, tend to its own recovery. This is best done during sleep.

NUTRITION

Nutrition is as vital to injury prevention as it is to triathlon training. As has been said elsewhere in this book, your body is an engine that needs fuel to function properly. Calories are fuel and your body needs a certain minimum each day to work. In addition, if your body does not get the correct nutrition, it will get increasingly tired. Not enough of the correct type of calories and you will begin the following day tired, unable to recover from the previous day's training session. Tiredness due to bad or insufficient nutrition will eventually contribute to an injury. See Chapter 9 (pages 75–85) for more on this subject.

PATIENCE IN REHAB

The mere mention of the word rehab to a triathlete is like mentioning Voldemort to a Harry Potter character! But the key to successful rehabilitation of an injury is *patience*.

It is one of the great contradictions of triathlon that the typical 'type A', gung-ho triathlete has to come to terms with performance gains being incremental, races being performed at a sustained and steady pace, and the inevitable occasional trip into rehab being under control of the dreaded patience. That, unfortunately, is triathlon reality.

Come back from injury rehab too early and you will probably make the injury worse. That, in turn, may lead to even longer in rehab, or even long-term damage to the offending muscle or injured body part. Patience in rehab, giving the injured body part enough time to completely heal, can even make it stronger than it was when it was injured.

CYCLING BIKE FIT

With the amount of hours put into training on the bike, and the stresses and strains that you will be putting your entire body under on the bike – from neck to back to quads to calves – taking the time to get the bike properly fitted will pay dividends. So make an appointment at a local bike shop that provides that service, or better yet a bike mechanic recommended by another cyclist you know, and have them fit your bike properly.

Once you have determined what your best position and angles are, mark everything clearly so that you can always return to those positions should you need to change them for any reason, such as when travelling and packing the bike into a travel case.

Cleats are another important element of bike fitting. If you look at the cleats and the undersole of your bike shoes, you can see there are different places the cleats can be screwed into the base. Changing the point where the cleats are attached to the sole of the shoe changes the angles and stresses on the muscles and body. It is surprising the difference it can make to comfort.

ICE BATHS

Under the category of 'No really, it does help!' comes ice baths. There is a reason that professionals and serious athletes swear by them, even though the first couple of minutes make you wish you were somewhere else.

Ice water immersion is thought to work better and have a more lasting effect on damaged muscles than simple ice packs, and it also cools large groups of muscles at the same time. Basically, an ice bath reduces tissue damage and swelling by constricting blood vessels. This also decreases metabolic activity. Getting out of the ice bath warms up the underlying tissues under the skin, promoting faster blood flow, which speeds up the disposal of damaged cells.

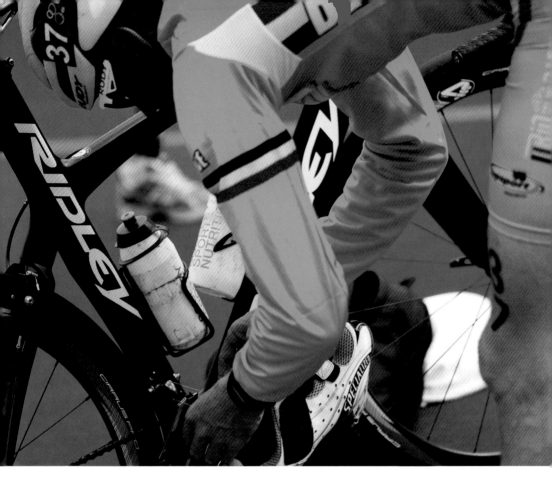

MASSAGE

A sports massage temporarily boosts blood circulation in areas on or under the skin, which then allows fresh nutrient-rich blood to rush back into that same area. The nurturing of nutrient-rich blood to an area can also speed up the rehabilitation of an injury. Massaging also helps push metabolic waste out of your system, such as lactic acid, and assist the body to pump blood to the heart.

Pain can also be relieved by the massaging of certain points on a muscle that feel both sensitive and tight, called trigger points.

CHECK EQUIPMENT REGULARLY

Equipment failure or malfunction is one of the main causes of injury for triathletes or endurance athletes, whether this entails a mechanical issue on the bike or ill-fitting or worn-out running shoes. The result is the same: injury immanent! The solution is to check equipment regularly, just as you would check basic levels on a car, like oil and brake fluid.

Preventive maintenance is also the best way to optimise performance from your equipment, as well as avoid injury to yourself. So schedule regular maintenance on your bike every week or two, perhaps the night before a regular Sunday long ride.

Also, keep track of the miles you have run in your running shoes, and if you run on consecutive days, rotate two pairs of the same shoe, if possible. When certain shoe rubbers get hot from running it can take them a long time to cool down and regain their original cushioning qualities.

That is not needed if you only run every other day, which is always a good preventive training schedule rule of thumb in any case: do not run on two consecutive days to save repetitive pounding wear and tear on your leg muscles, knees and joints.

OVERTRAINING

Overtraining is one of the main causes of injury in endurance athletes. In triathletes, it can be even worse as you try to get more and more training hours into the week in an effort to do enough for each of the three disciplines.

Overtraining repercussions often go hand-in-hand with inadequate nutrition, which leads to over-tiredness, lethargy, soreness and lack of strength, which in turn lead to bad technique and the inevitable injury as a consequence.

The standard rules apply: lots of recovery, pay attention to your nutrition, and listen to your body for any signs of overtiredness or soreness. In addition, if you are increasing your training volume, do not increase it by more than 10 per cent a week.

CONCLUSION

The best way to prevent injury in a masters athlete is to be proactive. As the body ages it will lose muscle and bone mass, strength and power will decline, VO2 max will decline, muscles and tendons will lose their elasticity and flexibility, and the body will take longer to recover from workouts and runs than it did when it was younger.

Knowing that, what is required is a custom training schedule tailored to the individual athlete, which allows for gradual build-up of workload. It also needs to include lots of recovery time, and extra sleep, to allow the body to rebuild and recharge.

Doing less in training as we age, with a more sedentary approach to training, is not necessary. Higher-intensity workouts, along with more focused training, but with extra precautions to allow the body to recover and a proactive approach to injury prevention, will allow an athlete to compete, and often increase performance, while at the same time maximising the possibilities of an injury-free season.

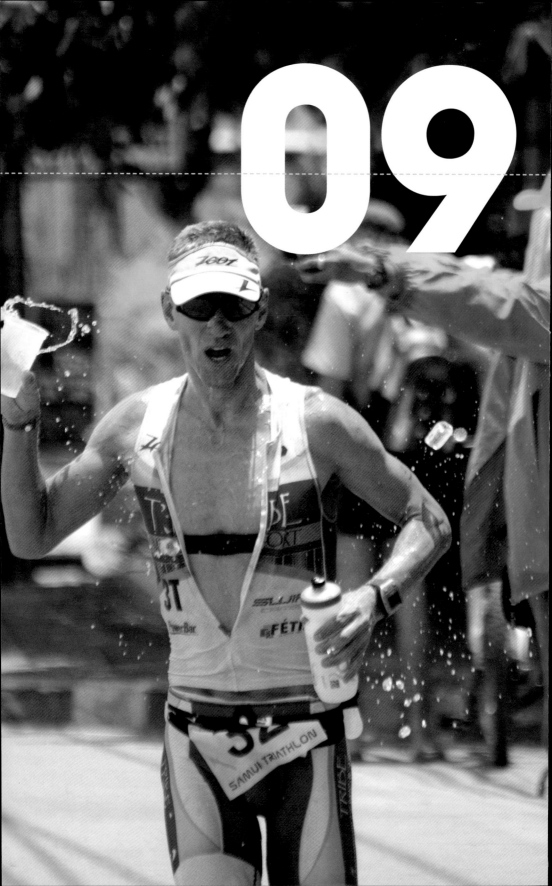

NUTRITION AND FUEL

THREE MASTERS CONSIDERATIONS DISCUSSED IN THIS CHAPTER:

- Diet equals energy. The older you get, the more important a balanced diet is to maintain energy, and therefore help fend off fatigue.
- The body is an engine; maintaining the correct daily calorie count, for both training and racing, ensures the engine can function optimally.
- Maintaining a daily food log helps keep track of both sufficient calories and the all-important balanced diet.

Proper nutrition is as fundamental a part of triathlon as putting in enough training mileage. You could even say it is a fourth discipline, to go along with swimming, running and cycling. Without the correct nutrition, the other three disciplines will not get you very far.

There have been thousands of books written about nutrition, and probably hundreds written about nutrition for athletes. However, it is one of the most overlooked fundamentals of the sport by triathletes themselves. Very few triathletes know all that they should know about correct nutrition and what to eat, and when, for optimum performance.

As mentioned elsewhere already in this book, in simple terms, the body is an engine and it needs the correct fuel, and enough of it, if it is to operate correctly. If it does not get it, performance not only suffers, but it can very quickly start to damage the body.

A BALANCED DIET

Generally speaking, when we talk of a good diet, what are we talking about? The first thing to consider is that a diet needs to be balanced. That means consuming a variety of foods from multiple different food groups, such as carbohydrates, protein, fruits and vegetables, dairy, even fats. Not all fats are bad, only some of them. The ones to avoid are saturated or trans fats.

The box below gives a short list of food examples of carbohydrates (the fastest energy supply for muscles), proteins (for building and rebuilding muscles) and fats (a more concentrated energy supply than carbohydrates). Like many foods, some of them do overlap categories.

- **Carbohydrates:** multi-grain bread, multi-grain bagels, rye crackers, bananas, oatmeal, brown rice, pasta, orange juice, non-fat yogurt, fruit, vegetables, whole grains.

- **Proteins:** Eggs, peanut butter on toast, turkey sandwich, spaghetti with meat sauce, lean red meat, skinless chicken, milk, fish (salmon, tuna, mackerel, swordfish – oily fish), beans, nuts, soy.

- **Fat (not saturated or trans):** avocado, fish, olive oil on salads, flaked almonds on granola, trail mix with nuts, vegetable oil.

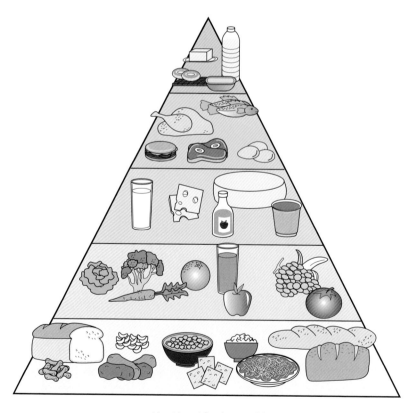

Nutritional food pyramid

A diet should include a full daily quota of vitamins and minerals. Some would say that if you have a correctly balanced diet then you should not need vitamin supplements. That may be true. However, who really has the time and resources to ensure the correct amount of vitamins are consumed every day directly from the food we consume? Unless you have a nutritionist available to analyse your diet, a convenient way to ensure enough vitamins each day is to simply take extra vitamin supplements.

Whatever side of the vitamin supplement argument you sit, just make sure you have the right amount of vitamins and minerals every day. One way of loading up on them is to eat fruit and vegetables. And yes, that includes broccoli and Brussels sprouts!

Also: fluids, fluids, fluids! Drink lots of fluids. It doesn't have to be straight water, though the higher the water content, the more hydrating it will be. But even some foods contribute to your water intake, especially fruit and salad vegetables, such as watermelon, cucumbers and tomatoes.

You can get in the habit of self-evaluating your hydration by checking the colour of your urine when you go to the bathroom. If it is darker or yellow, you should consume some more fluids. It should be almost clear in colour.

MAINTAIN THE CALORIE COUNT

The main factor in a balanced triathlon training diet is the amount of calories consumed. However, they should be good calories, rather than two hamburgers and a bucket of fried chicken!

We can go back to the engine analogy here. The human body is an engine, and an engine needs fuel to function. For the most part, calories are a body's fuel. Even a non-triathlon training body requires a certain amount of calories to function with enough energy each day.

As noted earlier, the best rule of thumb is to multiply your bodyweight in pounds by 14 and the total is the approximate amount of calories you need to consume each day to maintain your body weight, and not feel tired and energy-less the next day. For example, a woman weighing 9 stone 4 translates to $(14 \times 9) + 4 = 130$ pounds, so she would multiply 130×14 and come up with 1,820 calories a day that she needs to consume.

Another ballpark figure is to say anyone exercising or training will generally burn around 500 calories an hour more while they exercise than they would otherwise. For someone training at triathlon for 2 hours a day, that is an extra 1,000 calories they will burn, and will therefore have to consume.

So that same 130 pound woman, triathlon training for 2 hours a day, will need to consume something around 2,820 calories or so just to maintain her bodyweight (i.e. her 1,820 calories for the typical day without considering exercise, plus 1,000 calories for the 2 hours of training).

If you do not reach your target calorie intake each day, especially if you are training, two things will happen pretty quickly. The first is that in a day or two you will begin to feel extremely tired, sore and lethargic. That is because your body is being asked to function on insufficient amounts of fuel. The second thing that can happen is extremely detrimental to a triathlete. If your body is not getting enough calories (energy) by eating, it will look elsewhere for it. And that place will be the protein in the muscles. Yes, horror movie fans, your body will start to eat itself!

If you need to lose weight while exercising, you still need to consume enough calories for the body to function properly. So you need to get within 500 calories of your target calorie count each day. The rule is to lose weight gradually, not overnight. If you try to lose weight too fast, your training will suffer. If you ask the body to train with insufficient fuel, you increase the risk of injury.

THE TRIATHLETE'S DIET

So with regard to triathlon, what is the difference between a triathlete's balanced diet and the balanced diet of a more sane, normal person?

The main difference initially will be volume and balance of nutrients, which can change each day depending on training schedule, what you do that day, and workout session. As mentioned above, a triathlete will consume more calories. They will also consume more carbohydrates and protein. Longer training sessions, especially applicable for Ironman training, will require a lot more carbohydrates. Carbohydrates equate to energy in the body. Energy for carbohydrates is stored in the muscles as glycogen.

When you 'carbo load' before a race, for example with pasta, you stock up on glycogen, which is then used during the event. Temporarily increasing carbohydrates in the diet ensures that many of the extra calories being taken in are for race use. Stocking up on glycogen in the days before a race can delay the onset of muscle fatigue on race-day two-fold, or even three-fold.

Increasing temporary energy reserves and decreasing exercise in a taper just before the race should result in a highly energised body, well rested, and with a large stock of glycogen to call on.

So to restate the obvious, the first consideration of a diet is to consume enough food, and the right type of food, to meet the daily energy demands that are being placed on the body. Some days will be very different from the next, but many days will be similar. The energy demands of a 5-hour ride at the weekend will be very different from a 'brick' session of a 2-kilometre swim followed by an easy 5-kilometre run on the treadmill.

While you can have a general daily diet and nutrition plan, it needs to be flexible enough to encompass the many changes and variations of a triathlon training schedule.

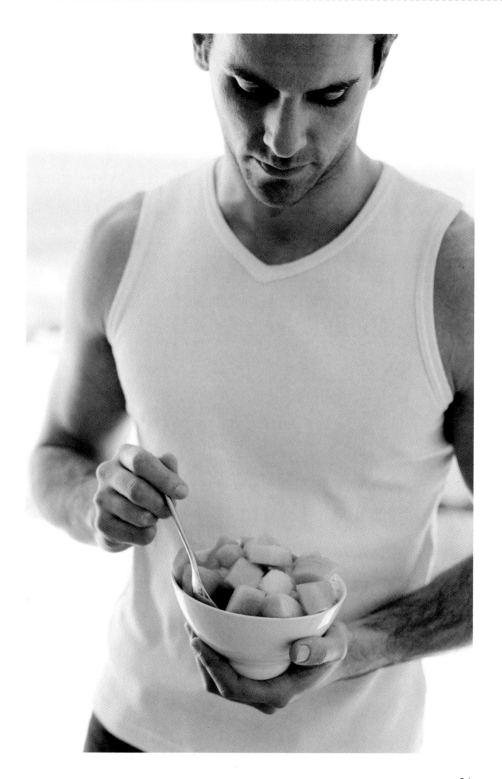

CONSUMING CALORIES

The first thing is to figure out exactly what you are doing today. Are you swimming, biking or running? Are you weight training in the gym? Are you doing a single discipline or are you doing a brick session of two or three disciplines right after the other? What is the duration of the training session and what are the intensity levels going to be? From the perspective of calorie intake, an easy 5-mile run that takes an hour is going to look very different from an hour of fast intervals in the pool.

In addition, intensity levels affect people in different ways. In fact, exercise affects people in different ways as well, in terms of what solids they can and cannot eat. Some people can't eat at all if they are undergoing a sustained high-intensity workout. Even gels are difficult for them to consume. That would be something to think about when choosing a race to compete in. Shorter triathlon races are inevitably of a much higher intensity level than longer races, such as half-Ironman distances. However, even shorter distance triathlons can take upwards of 2 hours to complete.

If you are not sure about what your body will let you eat at different intensity levels and distances, then one of the basic rules of triathlon applies: test out everything in training first. If you have trouble consuming solids, and even gels, then use trial and error with different foods, distances and intensities in training sessions. Also, try different brands of gel, energy drinks and energy bars. There are so many different bands and types; you could well find one that suits your constitution better than the others do.

Depending on your training schedule and workout, there might be a lot of calories to be taken in by the body in a single day. Just how should these calories be consumed?

EAT SMALLER MEALS MORE OFTEN

Instead of three large meals in a day, break it down into five or six smaller daily meals and snacks. Ideally, the calories/energy you consume with each meal or snack should be enough to fuel you for the next 2–3 hours, and no more. That way those calories get used up almost immediately. With bigger meals there is too much food to be used straight away, so what isn't used gets stored in the body as fat.

Although in these modern times it is increasingly difficult to avoid 'artificial' anything, avoiding 'unnatural' foods whenever you can is never a bad thing. That means avoiding fried foods and other foods that contain processed oils. However, olive oil and vegetable oils are a step in the right direction. Whenever possible, avoid artificial additives and preservatives as well, along with foods with added sugar and processed grains. Many people swear by organic foods generally, because they are meant to be grown naturally, with no chemicals or pesticides used in the growing process.

ADDITIONAL WORKOUT TIPS

A few special nutrition tips for workouts:

- Be sure to eat before a long-duration workout or a high-intensity workout. Not just before it starts, but an hour or two before to give your body some time to absorb some of the energy provided in the meal.

- A common benchmark workout time often used as to when to start refuelling is if a workout extends past 90 minutes. If anything, that is too long to wait. The rule of thumb should be to start hydrating as soon as you feel thirsty. On a hot day that may be 20 minutes into the workout, or even less. Do not put off rehydrating with either water or an enhanced sports drink if you feel the need. The same is true for solids or gels, although you are much more likely not to feel the need for something more solid than fluid until much longer into a workout.

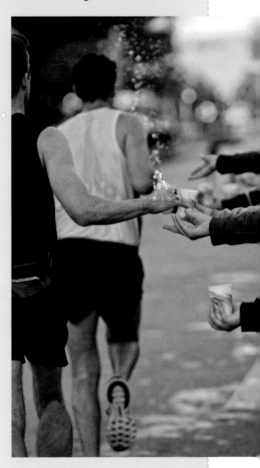

- A word of warning about thirst and the masters athlete. The older an athlete gets, the less frequent their thirst demands. That does not mean they require less fluids, it means that the demand for them is not registering like they would if they were younger. So a tip is to work out how much fluids need to be consumed every 15 minutes and drink that amount whether you feel thirsty or not.

- A ballpark figure is to consume around ¾ litre (24 oz) of fluids every hour on a day that is not hot. Break that down into roughly 175 ml every 15 minutes, and be sure to drink that amount. Once you get behind on fluid consumption it is difficult to catch up.

- After finishing a hard workout, consume a combination of carbohydrates (for muscle glycogen replacement), protein (to rebuild and repair muscles) and an electrolyte-enhanced drink (for hydration).

Something that is often overlooked when putting together nutrition plans is personal food preferences. We spend so much time eating, it stands to reason we should enjoy it. There are not many people that dislike eating, and some love it! In addition, everyone is different in what they like.

Initially, then, make a list of favourite foods. Find out which food category each falls into, what their nutrition make-up is, and try to include them in your nutrition plan.

KEEP A FOOD LOG

For the uninitiated, there is so much to keep track of with nutrition that it may seem daunting. What to eat, when to eat, how much to eat, and from which food groups? The best way to keep track of your nutrition needs, and what you have or have not done, is with a food log.

In its simplest form, each day write down what you have eaten. That way you can keep track of your calorie intake, and which food groups are best represented and which are not. As always, you are looking for a balanced diet, optimised for your triathlon training and needs.

A food log can also be used for planning your dietary requirements ahead of time. Once you know the upcoming week's training schedule, and the daily demands each workout will place on your body – for example, how long each session will last and whether it is high intensity or low intensity – you can then plan your diet for the week, based around your training energy needs.

Start by writing down everything you eat, and the quantities of each food, before you change your diet, to give you an idea of how you have been eating. That will probably come as a surprise with regard to the amount of calories you consume and the types of calories.

Once you have got into the habit of keeping a food log, it can become an indispensable training tool, and a fundamental element in obtaining peak performance and optimising your triathlon training.

PEAK PERFORMANCE

Talking of peak performance, what are the steps in obtaining it? We have already quickly gone over some of them. So let us recap.

First, consider all the practical, external elements that will influence diet. What type of training does the schedule call for? For example, high-intensity workouts will require a slightly different balance than low-intensity ones, especially if the low intensity is coupled with added mileage, as is typical for Ironman-type training.

The three most important elements that contribute to peak performance are the amount of food and drink that a triathlete consumes (and that combined they attain the necessary daily calorie targets), the combination of various food varieties (carbohydrate, protein, fat) that provide the required nutrient and energy mixture, and when you consume them (timing).

The old saying 'timing is everything' actually applies to triathlon nutrition plans as well! You need to know when to take on fluids so you don't become dehydrated or that you rehydrate properly. You need to know when to take on carbohydrates for energy, and protein and amino acids for muscle repair and growth (did I hear someone mention steak?).

To repeat, everyone is different. That especially applies to their nutrition requirements and preferences. One of the basic rules of triathlon already mentioned is to try something in training first when problems don't matter as much, before you include it in competition. The same is especially true of nutrition. If you want to try out new foods, products or nutrition combinations, do so in the off-season or in a base training phase, not the week before a race!

CONCLUSION

Nutrition is vital for all triathletes, especially for masters. As the body ages it places different demands on individuals, depending on a plethora of personal factors, not just athletic. Keeping a food log, at least until an athlete knows their typical daily intake of calories better, is especially useful for masters athletes. Certain aspects of the body that decline with age – for example, muscle mass and bone density – can also be mitigated with better and more focused nutrition intake.

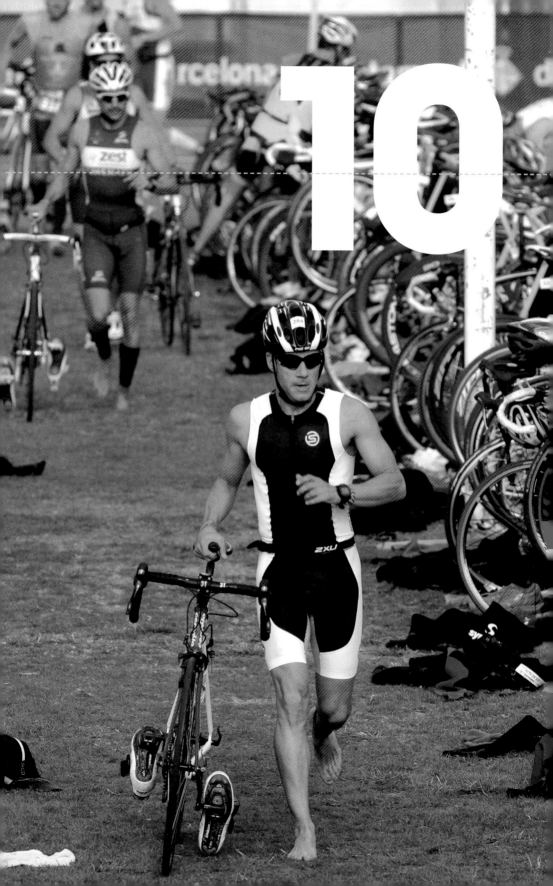

10

WHAT TRIATHLON GEAR IS REQUIRED?

THREE MASTERS CONSIDERATIONS DISCUSSED IN THIS CHAPTER:

- Choose comfort over speed when moving up from the beginner level, as you will be putting in a lot more training hours.

- Buy a road bike and not a triathlon bike initially as the angles on a tri bike are more extreme, and therefore more painful for long rides.

- It is vital for masters athletes to buy fresh running shoes every few months to help prevent running impact injuries.

Triathlon can be a rich person's sport. Perhaps that is one of the reasons that triathlon is becoming increasingly popular with masters athletes. Masters triathletes tend to have more disposable income at hand in their later years to spend.

However, the expensive equipment available – and the equipment that triathletes think they need to participate – is a far cry from what is actually needed to train and race.

This book is aimed at the enthusiastic masters post-beginner, who has dabbled in the sport a few hours a week and maybe raced a local sprint triathlon or two just to get their competitive feet wet, and is now looking to commit to it in a more serious way and move up to the intermediate level. As a result, they should already have enough equipment to be triathlon training and racing, at least at the beginner level.

The equipment described in this chapter is for the triathlete making the transition from beginner to advanced beginner or intermediate level. It is for the athlete who wants to learn more about the sport and needs to know what equipment is required to begin to train and race more seriously, and safely. Basically, this is a guideline list of equipment I wish someone had provided me with when I started the big move from beginner to intermediate.

BUYING FOR THREE DISCIPLINES

You need clothing and equipment for three different disciplines: swimming, cycling and running. Sometimes clothing and equipment overlaps, which is useful (and cheaper)! Unfortunately, often it does not. In addition, within those three disciplines, you have clothing and equipment for training, and then you have clothing and equipment for racing.

Sometimes the training and racing clothing and equipment also overlap, so that those items you use for training can also be used for racing. In addition, there is also recovery clothing, such as compression socks which many triathletes, and pro triathletes, also wear during the run as well as during recovery.

One word of warning: take care to check overlapping training/racing equipment carefully before a race as the repetitive use in training can cause mechanical malfunctions and additional wear and tear in equipment at the most inopportune time. The last thing anyone wants is for all the hard work of training to be negated because of a mechanical problem in the race.

WHAT IS YOUR COMMITMENT TO TRIATHLON?

There are always more questions in triathlon before you can provide an answer! Before you can start ticking off the clothing and equipment list, you need to revisit the evaluation questions already addressed earlier. For example, how serious are you at triathlon? How competitive do you want to be? How many hours a week do you want to spend in the saddle and in training? How much punishment are you prepared to put your body through in training, never mind the race? Do you favour comfort over speed?

If your ultimate goal is to really give your heart and soul to triathlon, to do whatever you can to be competitive, to improve your performance and to go as fast as you can in any race, whatever level that ends up being, then triathlon race clothing needs to be made for speed, and it should not be used for training. Instead, wear cheaper, easily replaceable (and probably more comfortable) clothing for training.

This is the minimum list of clothing and equipment I would expect a serious, enthusiastic triathlete to have. Believe me, you could write multiple books on the minutiae of clothing and equipment that *very* serious triathletes could elect to buy, and many do. However, for now, start with this as your minimum, because at some time in training or in a race, you will need them all.

SWIMMING
Swimsuit – pool training

The first is a day-to-day, thrash-it-to-pieces swimming suit for use in a chlorinated pool, at least twice a week (depending on your training schedule). If you can afford it, make this a tight fitting pool race suit/shorts that fit similar to your race tri shorts/suit, and not an old pair of board shorts hanging down by your knees like granny underwear! Chlorine in a swimming pool will destroy a tri suit (unless it is chlorine-resistant), so you need something relatively inexpensive that can take the chemicals and the punishment, week in, week out.

Swimsuit – open water/beach

If you have got a good training pair of shorts or suit for the pool (i.e. not cheap), then you probably don't want to run the risk of trashing them by swimming in a lake or off a beach. So get something that you don't mind messing up when you are swimming, when it's not a quality training swim. For men that might just be a pair of board shorts, or for women a cheap but robust swimsuit.

Race tri suit

Now we're talking! This is your speed suit. You only use this for racing. You might also use it a little for open water swim training, if you are not wearing a wetsuit, and in the pool a couple of weeks before your race to get the feel wearing it in the water. But other than that, it's probably going to be a lot more expensive than a regular swimming suit, so you really only want to break it out when you need to.

Super-duper tri suits come in two varieties: one, high-profile one-piece suits that really make you look like you know what you're doing; or two, separate matching tri shorts and tri top that still look and work great and are actually often more appropriate for warm weather swimming.

Wetsuit

In the real world, most people will be training and racing in temperatures that require a wetsuit in the water. However, you may not need a wetsuit at all, even for racing. If you have your upcoming season mapped out and you know the races you want to compete in are all warm enough for you not to wear a wetsuit, or are wetsuit-illegal (i.e. the water is too warm to wear one even if you wanted to according to triathlon rules), then save your money and spend it somewhere else. Believe me, there will be plenty to spend it on with triathlon! A good triathlon wetsuit can cost £150–250 ($250–400). Worst-case scenario is that you can rent that same suit, if you have to, for around £30–40 ($50–60) a week.

There are two main exceptions to that. First, if you are going to a race where you will wear one, you need to do some training in the same suit to get used to swimming in it. It is a very different feel compared with swimming without one. Second, you will definitely need to do some open water swim training, either in the ocean or in a lake. In most parts of the world, the ocean is cold enough for a wetsuit year round.

There is a third exception, but this is more of a tip. If you are not a strong swimmer, then you will probably want to use a wetsuit in a race whenever it is legal. When you swim, part of the physical effort you exert is keeping your hips up and your legs and back end of your body close to the surface. That alone can be tiring. A wetsuit will do that for you. As a result, most of the time, you will come out of a wetsuit swim feeling less tired than swimming without one. So if you are a weak swimmer, look to target races in your season where you know a wetsuit can be worn.

Wetsuit lubricant

Wetsuits are meant to be tight fitting – that's the whole point. They are like another layer of skin, only a more buoyant one that keeps you warmer. Getting them on can be a pain, but getting them off in the heat of competition can get crazy! So, apart from having your tri suit underneath, which will help you slide it off, use liberal portions of wetsuit lubricant. The less time you spend getting the suit off the better.

Swim goggles

A good pair of tight-fitting goggles are worth their weight in gold. However, do not have them so tight they give you a headache after 30 minutes in the pool. Try them first in the training pool, by leaving them on without moving them for at least the entire time of the intended race swim. If they fit and don't hurt, buy an identical second pair as a back-up! You should also buy a regular pair and then a pair that has anti-glare, tinted lenses for bright days. That will help in sighting the race course buoys in the swim, or when the sun rises in the sky.

Swimming cap

A swimming cap, usually colour-coded for the different age groups, will probably be provided by the race. However, you want to swim with two caps on during a race, so buy a tight-fitting one to wear underneath the race cap.

For races, put your own cap on first, then your goggles, and then the race-provided cap over the top of the goggle straps. In the mêlée of a triathlon swim start a second cap over your goggles will almost always prevent them from being knocked off your head and into the water if there is contact. And there is always contact in a triathlon swim!

In addition, some people like to train in swim caps, as they can be useful to keep long hair in check, as well as shaving seconds off your lap times.

Sunscreen

This goes in under swimming, but it applies to every discipline! Another tip is to put sunscreen on before you put your tri suit on for the race, not the other way around. Smearing sunscreen on after you put on your tri suit never works. A tri suit never stays in the same place during a race, so you end up with painful strips of sunburn where your suit has moved over a quarter of an inch! Not only that, but you can get sunburn through the clouds.

Towel

You will want two towels. One is a small drying towel for when you run into T1 to dry off your feet and clean off the sand before putting on socks and bike shoes. The second is an actual transition towel or mat that you lay down next to your bike with all your triathlon gear and clothing laid out on it. Then, as you come into the two transitions, your gear for the next discipline is already laid out for you. Some triathletes get the most colourful towel they can find to make their bike easier to spot from the hundreds around it during the chaos of the transition area in a race.

CYCLING
Bike

A good bike will be the biggest expenditure in your triathlon career. The question is which one.

Most people will select road-based triathlons as their chosen path, but do not rule out off-road mountain bike-based triathlons without giving them some thought. Off-road triathlons, represented for the most part by the Xterra brand, have a swim, a trail-based mountain bike ride and a trail run to finish. Lots of fun, lots of dirt, and certainly not for the faint-hearted. If you can only afford one bike, and love mountain biking, or you already have a mountain bike, give Xterra triathlons a try and see if you like it.

Most serious Xterra racers also have a road bike as well as a mountain bike. You can get a more consistent bike training workout on the road when you are in your base endurance phase of training. As a result, most Xterra riders do most of their basic endurance bike training on the road, and their technical bike handling on the mountain bike trails. When moving to their pre-season phase of training, they will switch to more mountain biking than road.

That said, I trained for years, and many thousands of miles, using a mountain bike on the road, but with slick tyres in the place of knobby tyres. It was a slightly harder workout than using a road bike with skinnier road tyres, but it did the job and was much more comfortable on my bad back at the time because of the more upright sitting position.

Assuming you are a soon-to-be committed road triathlete, the question is: what type of road bike? Triathlon-specific bikes are expensive. They have a different set-up than a regular road racing bike – the angle of the seated rider is more acute, for example, making it a more uncomfortable (but more aerodynamic) ride, and are really designed for going fast with as little wind resistance as possible.

As a result, not even the professionals will do all their training on a tri bike. Much of their training will be on a road racing bike, which is more comfortable over long rides for day-to-day training and is really better designed for handling hills and steep climbs.

If you can only afford one bike as you move up to your initial next level of commitment, buy as good a road racing carbon drop-handlebar bike as you can. That will be your bread-and-butter training bike, and social fun bike as well, while you move into the lower intermediate levels. Buy a good, solid pair of carbon clip-on aerobars that you attach to the handlebars and you are all set for years of triathlon training and racing.

Once you've thrashed the living daylights out of that bike for a couple of years, suffered the slings and arrows (and crashes) of a few competitive battles, gained some expert bike handling skills (fast downhill sections anybody?), and fine-tuned your body to the point of superhuman capability, then think about buying a good tri bike.

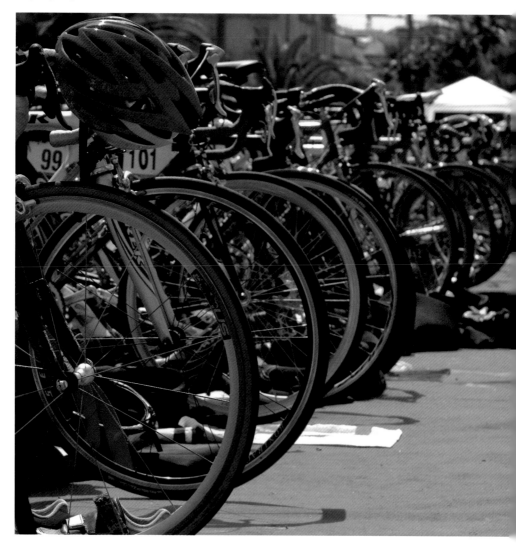

Generally speaking, a good carbon road racing bike (£1,200–2,500, or $2,000–4,000) will be cheaper than a good carbon tri bike (£1,800–5,000, or $3,000–8,000), so make sure you want to commit that sort of extra money to the triathlon cause.

Another tip, if you intend on going on group rides with non-tri riders who only have road bikes with drop handlebars: they will not like you turning up with a tri bike with aero handlebars and aerobars. Apart from the fact that most road bike riders are prejudiced against tri bike riders, they do have a point in that tri bikes do not necessarily handle as well as road bikes (although that is dependent on the skill of the rider, of course). Anyway, the point is that unless you are going on a group ride with fellow tri bike riders who have aerobars

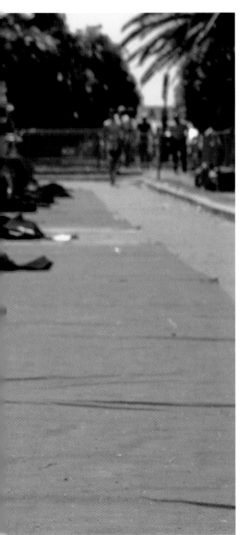

and aero handlebars, you should probably be riding a road bike with drop handlebars to avoid the drama that will ensue.

Bike shoes and clipless pedals

There are mountain bike shoes and road cycling shoes. For sure, you need a pair of bike shoes (and a pair of clipless pedals) if you want to improve your cycling skills and fitness, and your circular pedal stroke, with triathlon races as a goal.

Anyone who has visited an online cycling forum knows that any debate involving cycling equipment can go on ad infinitum, circle around and end up where it started!

The old argument of better stiffness and lighter weight with a road shoe compared with a mountain bike shoe really doesn't apply anymore. These days, you can get carbon shoes for road and off-road bikes. You can have stiffer mountain bike shoes than were available in the past.

Also, because of the deep tread on mountain bike shoes, which comes down below the cleats (which in turn slip into the pedal), you can walk properly in them, unlike road shoes where you have to waddle on your heels like a duck.

Stiff-soled road cycling shoes supposedly transfer more power to the pedals via smaller, more specifically designed cleats, while also helping to prevent numbed or cramping feet. But again, such results are as much hearsay as they are scientific and measurable.

That said, if you are buying a road bike, you are probably safest buying a pair of road shoes to go with it. You might even be able to haggle a free pair from the store you buy the bike from! But you have to negotiate. Unless you have a good reason to buy a pair of mountain bike shoes, buy a pair of road shoes.

The most important thing in buying any pair of shoes, whether for biking, running or walking, is comfort. Once you find a comfortable pair of shoes, buy them and move on to something that will make a real difference to your triathlon performance ... like training! Don't make drama where there is no drama!

Personally, I use the same pair of mountain bike shoes and pedals for every bike I ride. I have never had a situation where I thought that I could have gone faster on this road bike if I had been wearing a pair of road shoes instead of my favourite mountain bike shoes. I like a single pair of mountain bike shoes for all bikes because they are extremely comfortable; I can walk and run in them, and wherever I am and whatever bike I am riding, I only have to remember to bring one pair of shoes and pedals!

Ultimately, it comes down to personal preference. However, you wouldn't get a pro triathlete wearing a pair of mountain bike shoes at Kona! Why? One, their shoe sponsor would never let them. And two, if there is a marginal or infinitesimal difference in favour of a high-end road shoe over a high-end mountain bike shoe, then any pro is going to go for it because for them, it is the minutiae and seconds that count.

Helmet

Number one, you do not need an aero helmet! Number two, you do not need that high-end glossy helmet you saw in the magazine that retails for £200. What you do need is a solid bike helmet that is so comfortable on your head you don't know it's there. Bike helmets come certified as 'safe' by governing bodies, having obtained a minimum standard of quality and strength. If you want that peace of mind, look for a helmet with that standard displayed, and then you are good to go.

Cycling gloves

You absolutely need a good pair of padded cycling gloves! Anyone that has ever ridden a 70-mile hilly ride without them knows how indispensable they are, especially at around mile 50! Cycling gloves are cheap and well worth the money. Once you find a pair you like, buy two sets just so you know you always have them. They come in fingerless and full glove varieties, and it may be worth having both varieties available to suit the weather throughout the year.

Training cycling clothing

Training cycling clothing is not triathlon race clothing. You should not train in tri race clothing. Regular cycling shorts, for example, are more comfortable than tri shorts. Regular cycling shorts are more padded, and in addition, the chamois that you sit on is not designed for swimming in! With tri shorts the chamois is thinner and will dry quickly, as you will be riding in them immediately after you exit the water.

For training, you need padded cycling shorts, which come either as a one-piece 'bib' where the elastic straps attached to the actual shorts fit over your shoulders, or a separate pair of shorts that have a regular waistband. Again, it is a matter of personal preference. Anecdotally, bibs certainly seem to support the muscles in the legs and the back better than regular shorts. A down side is that they can only be used as cycling shorts and add another half layer of clothing above the waist on hot days.

Cycling tops come in short-sleeved and long-sleeved versions. Both have two or three pockets across the lower back for keeping necessary odds and ends in while you are on a ride (e.g. extra gel packets, inner tube, phone).

A thin, wind-proof and shower-proof jacket you can roll up and fit into a back cycling shirt pocket is extremely useful. It can often be taken on a ride instead of a long-sleeved cycling shirt, but also worn over the top of a long-sleeved shirt as well.

Water bottle

For both cycling training and run training, you will need water bottles. Minimum fluid intake should be around 750ml of fluids every hour. On a hot day, it can easily be twice that. You will need bottles for cycling in the race, but could well get away without the need for bottles in a shorter running race (5K and maybe 10K). In longer running races (over 10K), there will probably be aid stations every mile or so.

Efficient and constant hydration is one of the cornerstones of successful triathlon. Do not leave anything to chance, such as guessing your fluid intake during a race, that there will be an aid station when you need fluids, or even assuming there will be fluids at an aid station when you stop at one. There are numerous instances of latter-stage race aid stations running out of water on hot days because they have all been used up by earlier competitors rehydrating. Most serious triathletes will either be carrying a small water bottle with them on the run or, more likely, they will have a hydration belt around their waist with open-top pouches on that hold two or three small plastic bottles, or a larger regular bottle.

Be warned: having an aid station every mile sounds okay, but on a hot day that can be a long way before you get water. For example, even if you can complete a marathon in 4 hours 20 minutes, that only equates to running

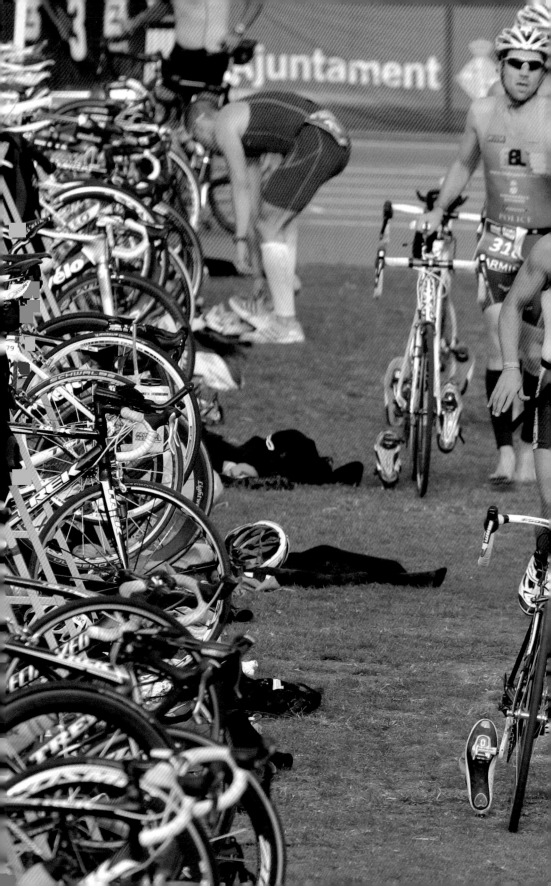

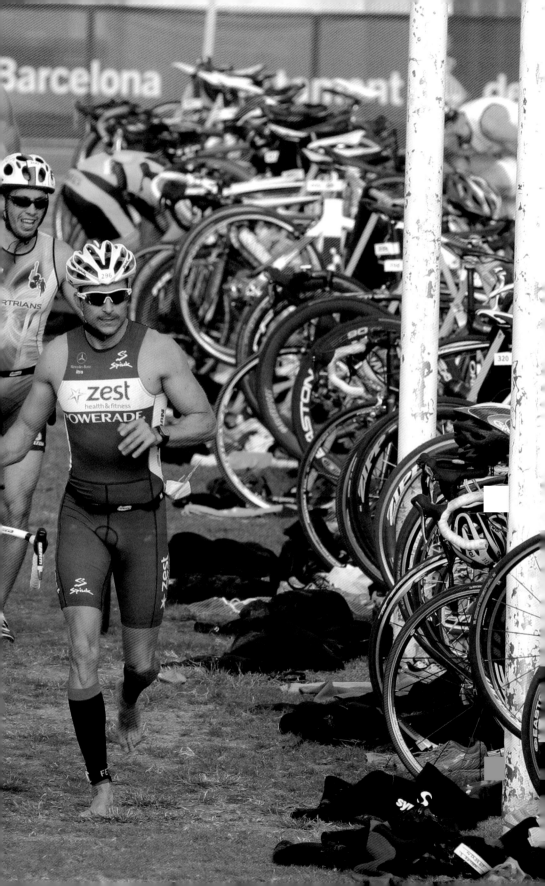

a mile in 10 minutes. That is 10 minutes between aid stations. When your body tells you it needs water, it should be given water. Never deny your body what it tells you it needs from a hydration or nutrition standpoint. Your body knows best.

Sport sunglasses

Close-fitting sport sunglasses are a must, and not just for sunny days. To prevent eye injuries they should be used in training all the time on both the run, but especially, the bike. Protect your eyes from glare, dust and the wind. The more training you do, the more important they become. And the same backup rule applies to sport sunglasses as pool goggles. When you find a pair you like and that fit perfectly, buy two pairs! It is not a question of *if* you break or lose your sunglasses, it is a question of *when*!

Race number belt

Although not essential, a race number belt is definitely useful in races as it saves valuable seconds in transition. These elastic belts allow a race number to be fixed quickly at the waist, and turned if needed from back to front and vice versa, instead of pinning the number to an item of clothing using safety pins.

Under saddle bag

This is an indispensable piece of equipment for cycling, both in racing and in training, but especially the latter. An under saddle bag may contain such basic repair tools as tyre levers, a small tyre pump, a CO_2 cartridge, a new inner tube, a chain repair tool, allen keys and, if you are 'old school', a puncture repair kit. The alternative is to fill up your cycling jersey pockets with repair tools and equipment. In the race that is not even an option, because cycling jerseys are not worn in triathlon races, just a tri suit or tri top. Having all the basic cycling repair and puncture tools already packed and fixed under the saddle in a flat pack gives piece of mind before embarking on a training ride, or a race.

RUNNING
Running Shoes

The most important part of any triathlete's list of equipment, at least from an injury prevention perspective, is a well-fitting, comfortable pair of running shoes.

Do not start training for a triathlon in a beat-up, 4-year-old pair of stinky tennis shoes that invariably have worn-out tread and no cushioning, even supposing they were specifically fitted for your own feet in the first place (which they almost certainly were not).

You should be running in a properly fitted pair of running shoes from day one. The most common injury in triathlon is repetitive motion injury. And the most common repetitive injury comes as a result of running. No matter how careful you are in building up your running in gradual increments of both volume and intensity, if you are wearing the wrong shoes, not designed for your type of feet, or with insufficient cushioning, you will get injured eventually.

One of the first purchases for a triathlete, no matter how serious they are, is a good pair of running shoes. For those who want to save seconds in transition, you can even buy running shoes with Velcro straps instead of laces or with special elastic or locking laces so you don't have to tie them.

Socks
Specifically designed sweat-repelling running socks that are comfortable and help keep you dry are a necessity, especially in hot climates – and especially if you intend to put in many hours of running a week. Do not buy 100 per cent cotton socks as they will stay wet and cause blisters in the summer, and keep you cold in the winter. Socks made with synthetic wicking materials are best. Personal preference comes into play again. Do you like thin lightweight socks when you run, or thicker, highly cushioned socks? Either way, buy your socks before you choose your running shoes as you will want to try on your new shoes in the store with the socks you will be using on your runs.

Running shorts and shirt
Modern-day wicking clothing takes sweat away from your body so you stay drier, even while you sweat, and it helps cool you down in the heat. A specially designed wicking running shirt, coupled with a loose-fitting, lightweight pair of actual running shorts, rather than regular gym shorts or heavier shorts from a different sport, represents a good early purchase. Don't forget this is your training clothing, because on race day, you will wear the same tri suit for all three disciplines.

Running hat
If you are training and racing where there is heat and sunshine, you should use some sort of a hat or visor. Even in colder climates, a running hat will keep sweat out of your eyes as you run, while also keeping your head warm and preventing body heat escaping out of the top of your head. As much as one third of a person's body heat escapes out the top of the head.

Coupled with a pair of sport sunglasses, a lightweight running hat with visor will prevent glare from affecting your eyes and will shield your eyes from the sun.

One of the biggest advantages of a baseball-style running hat on a hot race day, though, is that you can put ice under your hat from the aid stations to help cool you down and have it incrementally melt as you run.

ELECTRONICS
Heart rate monitor
A heart rate monitor has become very much a basic and inexpensive tool of triathletes, as well as endurance athletes generally. In its simplest form, an electronic device fixed to an elastic band around the chest reads the heart rate and sends it to a display on the athlete's wrist. The athlete can then equate an exact heart rate with the effort they are exerting and how hard their current session is.

Bike computer
Bike computers have become staple bike equipment for triathletes. Any serious triathlete, at whatever level, will need to have some way of learning to maintain a consistent speed. A bike computer does that. Unlike a Garmin, which works from GPS (see below), a simple bike computer has a readout display that fixes to the handlebars and works with a small magnetic device attached to the front wheel. That allows for the display of such data as current speed and average speed. More data can be provided according to the complexity, and cost, of the device.

Digital sports watch
A very useful and cheap electronic triathlon tool is a digital sports watch that acts as not only a regular watch, but also a stopwatch and lap counter. The lap counter feature will also be likely to allow you to split up the screen to show current lap time and overall current session time concurrently. The split-screen feature is useful for both racing, where you can see your time in each discipline separately, and for interval training, where you want to compare lap times within the same discipline.

Garmin-type device
A Garmin is a GPS-enabled electronic device that can provide real-time running, cycling and swimming data. GPS-enabled devices are aimed primarily at runners and triathletes, and can accurately measure distance covered, speed, time, altitude and even heart rate. They are expensive, and are definitely a question of personal preference. Some athletes feel they can deliver too much data, while many people swear by them. That said, just because the data is available does not mean you have to be a slave to it.

However, triathlon is all about consistency, and utilising just the 'current pace' feature while running will give you real time data that can prove invaluable when trying to maintain or when teaching your body to recognise a consistent pace.

OTHER
Sports drinks and race food
We have already discussed nutrition in the previous chapter, but it cannot be emphasised enough that without correct nutrition, you will be lucky to complete a triathlon, and you will certainly struggle with triathlon training.

Triathlon bag
A good triathlon bag can also double as a swim bag in training because it has different compartments for wet and dry clothes, so you can separate a wet swimsuit, wetsuit and damp towel from the rest of your dry gear. It will also often have extra-strong, but easily accessible hard-sided or cushioned compartments for sunglasses and fragile electronics. It can also be used as a useful gym and training bag year-round as well.

CONCLUSION

The list of triathlon equipment and clothing that a triathlete uses can be long and expensive, or it can be the minimum and reasonably priced. However, what clothing and equipment you buy is based on the answers to a number of questions concerning commitment to the sport – for example, the amount of training and how competitive you intend to be.

Masters athletes, though, also need to take into account that as they age they become more prone to injuries and repetitive motion damage to their ligaments, muscles, tendons and joints. As a result, favouring clothing and equipment that can provide extra cushioning and protection for the body can help maintain an injury-free training environment.

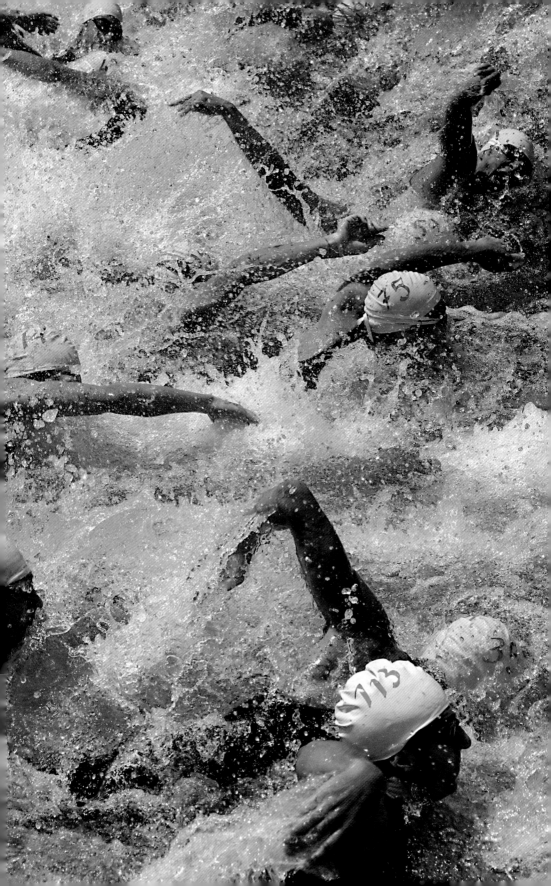

PART TWO

TRAINING AND RACING

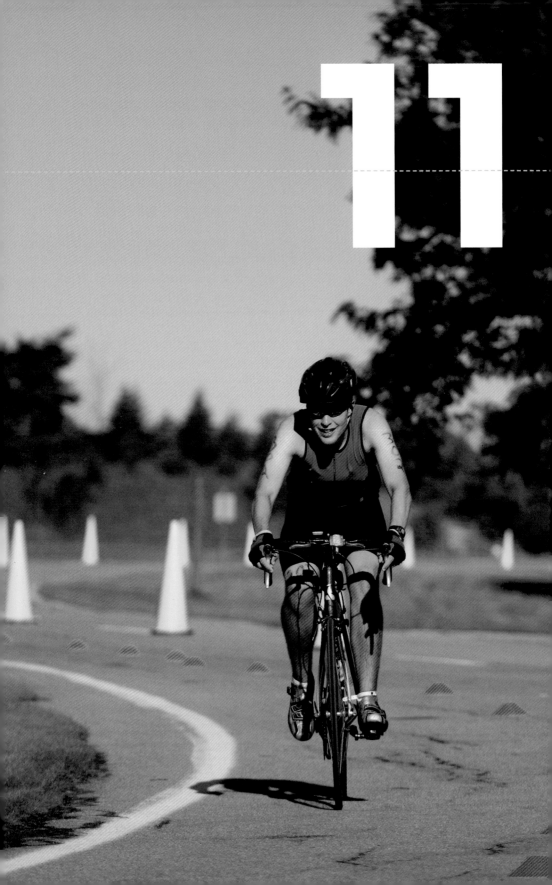

11

HIGH AND LOW INTENSITIES

A much-debated subject in triathlon training is intensity level. Are moderate, below-race-pace, low-intensity, but high-volume workouts the best, because they increase aerobic stamina at a reduced risk of injuries? Or should workouts be higher in intensity and lower in volume?

There are few training issues in triathlon that will cause such an impassioned response as the subject of high intensity versus low intensity. Every coach and athlete has their views about the benefits and the negatives, and few are the same.

HIGH INTENSITY VERSUS LOW INTENSITY

The fact is that whether you are a seasoned pro triathlete or new to the sport, you will spend much of your time doing low-intensity, high-volume training. Low-intensity, high-volume builds aerobic capacity at minimum risk of injury. If an athlete trained at high intensity all of the time, it would not be long before their body started to give out.

Not only that, but a body also needs to learn how to obtain energy from stored fat (read low-intensity, high-volume) and not just carbohydrates (read high intensity).

It takes more oxygen to burn fat than carbohydrates. As a result, as a body exercises harder and less oxygen is available, the body turns from fat to carbohydrates for energy. A rule of thumb as to when that handover actually happens is that if you are breathing hard and your muscles are starting to burn, then you are using carbohydrates for energy production and not fat. Below that physical exertion level, you are burning fat.

There is a benefit to the triathlete. As a result, the fitter you are, the longer you can rely on fat for energy before diminished oxygen supplies necessitate the move to carbohydrates, which are in more limited supply than fat.

While many believe that the best way to build a triathlon base is through low-intensity, long-distance training sessions, the reality is that a combination of both low and high intensities is necessary. This aerobic development helps in our ability to utilise stored fat in the body to create energy, adding to both our endurance and physiological efficiency.

HIGH INTENSITY COMBATS PHYSICAL DECLINE

In addition, in masters athletes, there are additional reasons for high-intensity training, as described elsewhere in this book. In the first place, it slows down the VO_2 max decline in older athletes; in addition, it helps maintain the fast-twitch muscle fibres, which decline with age and result in slower reaction times and explosive, sprinting abilities. A third reason is that high-intensity training helps build mitochondria cells in muscles, a topic discussed in more detail later in this chapter.

There are no quick fixes in triathlon training. The maximum performance gains are through consistent and increasingly progressive training. Consistency is the key. However, anyone who trains at the same intensity for weeks, or even months, at a time will eventually show little performance improvement. Whether it is swimming, cycling, running or strength training, the body shows the best performance improvement as a result of a mixture of intensity levels and progressively hard training, followed by a recovery period for the muscles to rebuild.

Although low intensity generally means the use of fat in the process of creating energy, and not carbohydrates, everyone is different as to when that change-over occurs. Level of fitness plays a large role in determining at what point someone will switch to carbohydrates to produce energy and not fat. Because everyone has only a limited supply of carbohydrates, the goal is to maximise efficiency and effort, while utilising fat for energy as long as possible before moving on to carbohydrates. Diet and fatigue also play a part in determining at what point someone makes that change.

While an athlete is in their off-season, in their base endurance phase and getting the body ready to accept greater training loads, most of the training should be at low intensity, but still with some higher-intensity sessions.

High-intensity training burns up more calories than low-intensity training. It does this because more energy, increased blood flow and more muscles are used, and with greater intensity. As a result, your post-exercise metabolism also gets higher and stays at a higher level for longer, the harder and faster you exercise during your training session. The result is that you keep burning calories through the day. This enhances oxygen and nutrient delivery to the muscles of the body, as well as increasing blood vessel capillarisation and mitochondrial density.

MITOCHONDRIA ARE THE BODY'S POWER PLANTS

Mitochondria are the power plants of the body's muscle and other cells, which utilise both oxygen and glucose to produce adenosine triphosphate (ATP). New mitochondria grow in the muscles used as a result of endurance training, which in turn improves endurance by allowing those same muscles to be better fuelled aerobically. Essentially, they help convert fat, glucose and protein into usable energy.

A great deal of prevailing thought contends that the growth of essential energy processing mitochondria is optimised under high intensity exercise, with short intervals approaching VO_2 max or greater. Creating larger and more plentiful mitochondria in the muscle cells essentially lets you go faster before reaching your lactate threshold. It also allows you to recover from lactate build-up workouts more quickly.

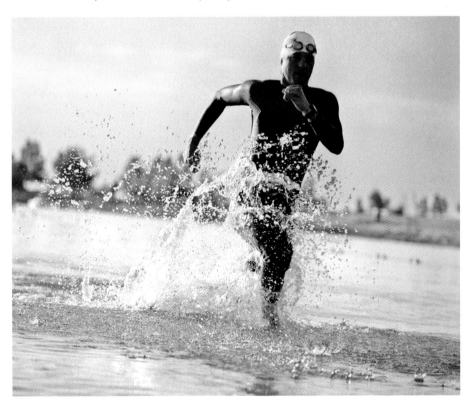

While it is possible to increase mitochondria from long, low-intensity training sessions, there comes a point where volume alone (i.e. without high intensity) will not boost mitochondrial density. Chalk another one up for high intensity.

HIGH-INTENSITY RECOVERY AND THE MENTAL STATE

A triathlete's body needs to be trained to utilise both fat and carbohydrates for energy. For longer triathlons, it is essential that fat is utilised for energy. In training, a body should be encouraged to conserve energy, not use it. As a result, training sessions should be planned so both fat and carbohydrates are used.

A good rule of thumb is that if you are breathing hard and your muscles are burning, you are utilising carbohydrates. If you are below that exertion and can even hold a conversation, then you are utilising fat stores for energy. The fitter you are, the more your body can rely on fat at the lower-to-medium endurance paces.

There are practical race considerations, as well as physiological. High-intensity training sessions, or high-intensity sections of workouts, help train an athlete to increase their pace and effort if needed, such as when overtaking, hill climbing or sprinting for the finish. However, there is also a need to also practise recovering from such high-intensity efforts during the race. It is no good putting in a great effort to pass a rider up a hill only to have to slow down and recover on the other side, allowing them to catch up again.

The reality of high-intensity training is that it is very tough, and it will eventually take its mental toll of the athlete. The mental state of the athlete has to be taken into consideration at some point. Anyone subjected to month after month of high-intensity training will eventually have to deal with such mental factors as motivation. Athletes can burn out very quickly on high-intensity training, even professional triathletes. Knowing that, day after day, you are going to punish your body with painful, high-intensity training will inevitably be a cause for concern for any athlete, and for their coach.

TRAINING TIME AND INTENSITY LEVELS

How much time the athlete has to train can also become a factor when choosing between low- and high-intensity training schedules. If you are an advocate of low-intensity, high-volume training, and yet only have 6 hours to train a week, that is not going to work. If that is the case, season goals will probably have to be re-evaluated, with future competitions focused on sprint races, and then a focus on high intensity training can be applied with those goals in mind.

Quite often, an athlete is not in a position to set up a season-long training schedule, with set race goals, in advance. Instead, work or other pressing matters dictate that they must be flexible enough to change their schedule at a few days' notice.

The debate between high-intensity, low-volume and low-intensity, high-volume in swimming is often even more contentious. In swimming, high-intensity advocates are also up against an embedded training culture that believes it takes hundreds of hours in the pool to achieve the right stroke 'feel', as well as technique and efficiency.

However, critics of that argument contend that high-volume training depletes the glycogen stored in the muscles, which carbohydrates access, as well as adding to the fatigue of the fast-twitch muscle fibres by reducing their force production, which many short swim race distances utilise. That is probably why tapering is so important for swimmers who have engaged in high-volume training, because it probably allows the fast-twitch fibres to regain their high-velocity properties. Basically, the shorter a swimming race – anything under 2 minutes – the more a body's anaerobic energy system comes into play, while the longer the race, the greater the role of the aerobic energy system.

Of course, there is low intensity and high intensity, and everything in-between. Certainly, you are not going to hold a high-intensity running pace for very long. The same can be said for swimming in the pool, or riding the bike. As a result, there are different levels of intensity.

Quite often this is represented by a number scale – from one to twenty, for example, with one being extremely easy and twenty being as hard as you can go. These numbers are then matched with target heart rates – such as easy, medium, tempo and hard.

CONCLUSION

Like much of triathlon, there are multiple arguments for any given subject, and multiple answers that can seem to work, because everyone is different in their physical and mental make-up. However, what works for one person may not work for another person of the same age, weight and body type. This is complicated by age, of course, because everyone ages in different ways and at different speeds.

Suffice it to say that there is a need to look on the 'low-intensity, high-volume' versus 'high-intensity, low-volume' debate as a balanced diet. You need both, but in different portions, and at different times of the year, depending on your training and racing schedule as well as your physical and mental make-up. Again, chalk up another reason to use customised training schedules and not off-the-shelf programmes.

From a masters perspective, that is especially true as high-intensity workouts help to mitigate VO2 max decline, muscle and bone mass deterioration, and enhance mitochondria cell production in muscles.

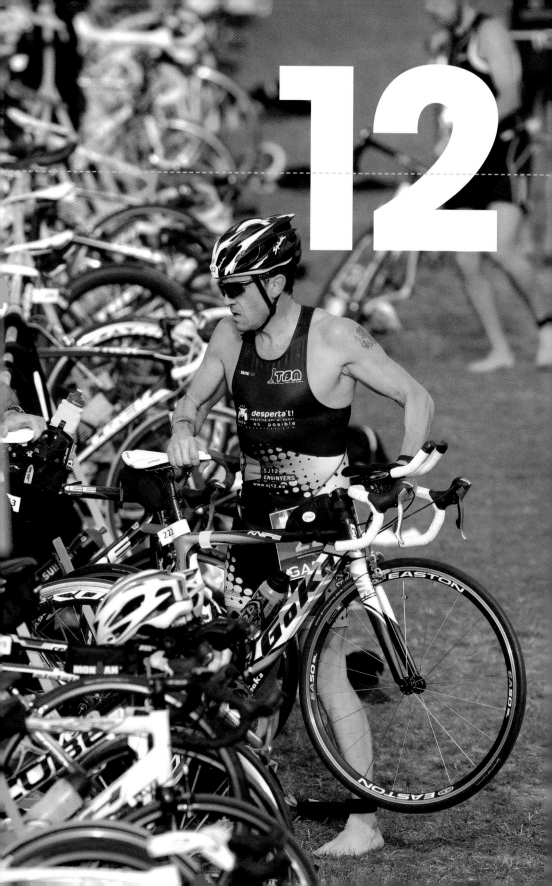

12

ONE SPORT, BUT THREE DISCIPLINES

Triathlon training and racing is all about managing the inter-relationships between the three athletic disciplines of the sport: swimming, cycling and running. What many triathletes do not fully comprehend is that those three disciplines do not exist in isolation from each other. The triathlete always needs to train in one discipline with the other two in mind. In addition, complicating the issue is the age of the athlete.

For example, in its simplest form, the swim needs to be completed using predominantly the arms and upper body, and as little leg muscle power as possible. That is because once the swim is completed, the arms are essentially unused for the rest of the triathlon. The bike section has to then be completed in such a way that it taxes the running muscles as little as possible. The key to triathlon success is the ability of the triathlete to post a strong, steady run on tired leg muscles.

While there are three distinct and separate disciplines, a triathlete cannot train as though they are separate. Often it is necessary to go easier in swimming or biking, because energy has to be saved for the run.

DO NOT TRAIN LIKE IT IS THREE INDEPENDENT SPORTS

As mentioned, triathlon is a single sport consisting of three separate disciplines. Many triathletes come to triathlon from single sports – swimming, cycling or running – and think that the way to approach training is to focus on each discipline separately and train for each as if it were a separate sport. That approach will not work successfully with triathlon.

In the first place, the training time involved would be too great. Triathletes, having to train for three events instead of one, will always be lacking in training hours for each discipline compared with a single-sport athlete.

For a triathlete training in the pool two or three times a week, for example, focus has to be placed on endurance, stamina, some speed, strength, motor skills and basic technique to maximise efficiency. As a result, they will have to prioritise their swimming needs, just as they have to prioritise their training to address their biggest athletic shortcomings first. A single-sport swimmer has plenty of days and sessions to address them, whereas the triathlete, with three disciplines instead of one, does not.

In addition, the triathlete then has to adapt pool technique to open water technique and, in the case of an Ironman mass start, the 2,000 other bodies all vying for the same stretch of clear water as them!

Secondly, and more importantly, it is not three separate events. Instead, it is the combination of swimming, cycling and running. Only the combined times of all three events matter in the end. Individual discipline excellence means very little if the other two disciplines are severely lacking. Triathlon success is a balance between the three disciplines.

Often, a workout will consist of a 'brick' session, where training for two of the disciplines is accomplished back-to-back, just as in a race – for example, a run immediately following a ride, or a ride immediately following a swim.

A triathlete has to train and race each of the three disciplines in relation to the other two. As a result, in triathlon there are some differences in how each event is performed over how they would be performed as a single sport.

In short, in triathlon the swim is executed mainly using the upper body, with a balance between speed, efficiency and maximum energy savings for the remainder of the race. The bike section is performed with the run in mind, utilising muscles and technique that fatigue the run muscles the least. In addition, because the run is performed at the end of an already taxing race, the approach to the run is inevitably different than if you start the run with fresh legs.

DON'T FOCUS ON YOUR STRONGEST EVENT

It is only human nature to focus on what makes us look the best, or that we enjoy doing the most. However, in triathlon that is a recipe for mediocrity. Most athletes come to triathlon from a single sport, which is invariably the sport they are good at, be it swimming, cycling or running. While, both psychologically and physically, that can be a benefit and big boost to morale during training and racing, to focus on what is already a personal strength is counter-productive.

In terms of triathlon training, you do not want to focus mainly on your strongest discipline, nor allocate your training time equally between the three events.

If you have a particular strength, for example the run, while it is good in that you know you are finishing with your best event, your main time improvements for a triathlon will not come from improvements in that discipline, because it is already a strong discipline for you.

FOCUS ON WEAKEST DISCIPLINE FOR MAXIMUM TIME GAINS

As a result, you need to focus more on your weakest discipline, or the two weakest disciplines. That does not mean ignoring training in your strongest discipline. You should. If it is your strength event, you want to maintain it as such. However, the best opportunity to find overall time improvements lies with your weakest discipline.

If cycling is your weakest discipline, for example, initial technique training followed by a sizable portion of your training schedule devoted to cycling endurance and putting in hours on the road will almost certainly result in considerable overall triathlon time improvements. You will spend most of your time in any triathlon race on the bike, so any major performance improvement in that discipline will reflect in considerable overall performance gains.

However, while most triathletes' weakest event will be swimming, that will probably be the shortest of the three disciplines during a race. In swimming, faster and stronger in stroke technique rarely means quicker for the average age-grouper. In swimming, technique is everything. Improve technique and you will get quicker, whether endurance improves in the water or not.

In triathlon swimming, though, unlike regular swimming, you are also trying to maximise efficiency and speed in the water with a minimum of effort, so a leg kick is barely used. It is predominantly upper body, because the legs will be used for the rest of the triathlon, whereas the arms will not. That technique is very different from regular swimming. Most triathletes will use their legs mainly for stability and to help raise the hips up in order to make the body more streamlined in the water, and therefore more efficient.

ALL DISCIPLINES ARE NOT CREATED EQUAL

A word of caution though – all disciplines are not created equal.

Swimming, as mentioned, is a small part of a triathlon race. Cycling will be the longest part of a race, and running second longest. Swimming may only represent as little as a seventh or an eighth of a triathlon race time, and

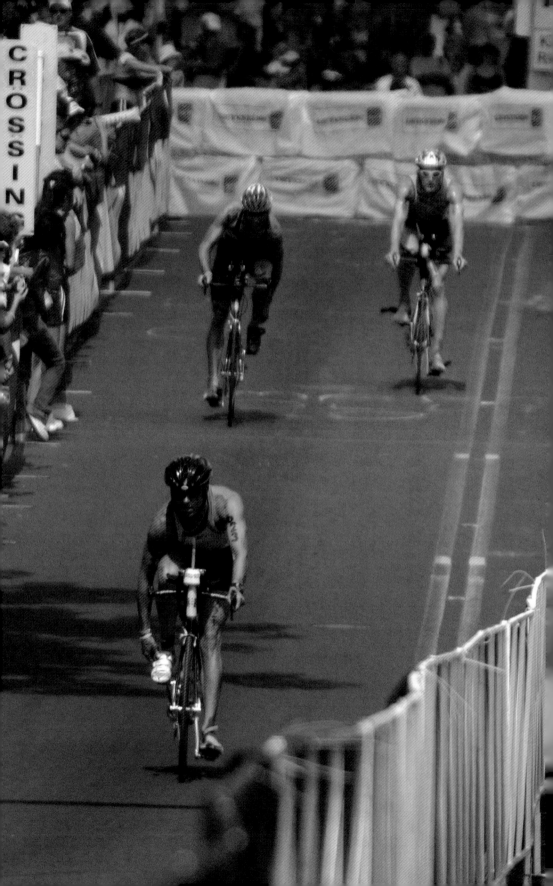

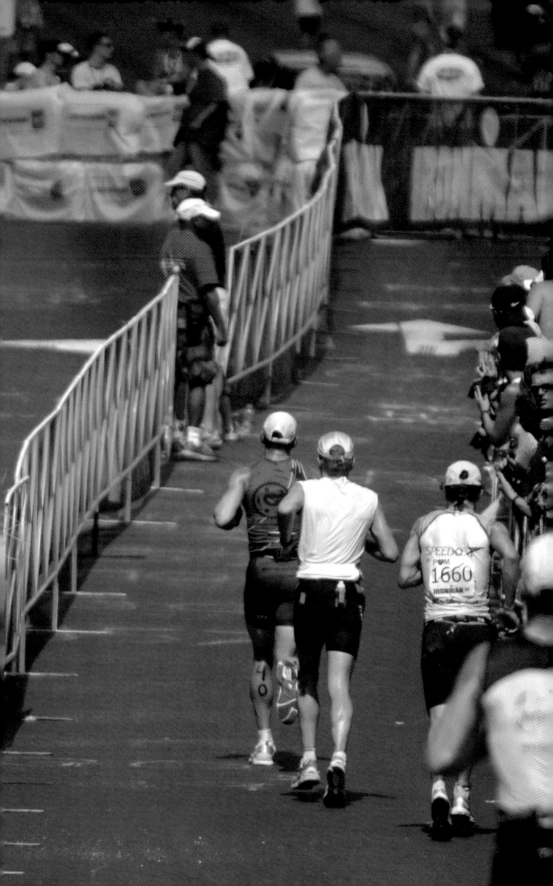

perhaps even less. As a result, it makes no sense to spend a third of all your training time at swim practice. The triathlon improvement returns will not reflect the hours spent in the pool. This is not the sport of swimming. Instead, it is the sport of triathlon, which incorporates swimming as the first of its three disciplines.

For the weaker swimmer, though, the emphasis is to complete the swim in an efficient manner, with minimum negative fatigue impact on the body. As a result, swim sessions should be shorter rather than longer, emphasising correct technique. They should be shorter, but there should be more of them.

Why? Because at the outset in triathlon training, correct swim technique is paramount. However, correct technique will invariably break down as fatigue sets in after a few hundred yards or so in the pool. So keep the swim training session, or the individual workouts within that training session, short enough to allow correct technique to be used at all times before fatigue sets in. Instead of two longer swim training sessions a week, incorporate three or four shorter sessions, where the emphasis is on correct, efficient technique. Then, once correct technique can be maintained, reduce the number of swim workouts, but make each one longer.

The biggest improvement in triathlon performance comes from a balanced approach to training, focused on an intended balanced race performance. On an individual level, once correct technique has been obtained in all three events, tailoring training to improve the weakest events will almost certainly result in the biggest overall performance time improvement.

However, what also needs to be considered is how big a part of the race that discipline represents in terms of time. For example, in an Ironman race, coming out of the swim, many fit, intermediate age-groupers will be only 30 minutes behind the professionals. By the end of the Ironman race, though, the gap to the winning pro will have widened to over 4 hours!

THE DIFFERENCE BETWEEN TRIATHLON AND NON-TRIATHLON RUNNING AND CYCLING

For longer triathlons like Ironman and half-Ironman, one difference between triathlon running and normal running, and triathlon cycling and normal cycling, is that with triathlon running, you begin the run with tired muscles and fatigue well established in the body. As a result, a triathlete needs to tax the run muscles as little as possible on the cycling leg, while still maintaining a competitive speed.

The endlessly debated question in triathlon is how you actually change cycling and running technique to reflect that. Or do you change it at all?

With a triathlon race, the triathlete is ultimately running on fatigued legs, even at the start of the run segment. Inevitably, that will likely mean reduced stride length and lower range of motion.

One school of thought argues that, as a result, a triathlete needs to train to run at a shorter stride length, but at a higher cadence, in order to maintain speed and lessen leg fatigue. That requires fast-twitch muscles. It also means running with lower knee lift and back lift in order to use less energy and be more efficient. However, that in turn will mean a higher heart rate.

As a result, so the argument goes, there is a need to conserve those fast-twitch muscles on the ride and keep heart rate lower. Therefore, you need to ride at a lower cadence (because a high cadence will use the same fast-twitch muscles) with bigger gears, which also lowers heart rate and offers high efficiency. Lower heart rate and cadence means that the body can utilise fat for energy instead of the more oxygen-dependent carbohydrates, which will be used on the run.

With triathlon cycling, then, the key is completing the bike leg with as little aerobic fatigue as possible in the muscles, which will then be used on the run.

In triathlon, training on the bike is conducted with the knowledge that there is a run, and usually a long run, to follow. While the triathlon cycling emphasis is on endurance, lactate tolerance and strength, the regular cycling training goals would also include group riding, acceleration and speed.

Because, with triathlon, the run begins with already fatigued and taxed muscles, fatigue will set in much quicker than with single-sport runners. The key then is really in the lead-up to the run, and saving the muscles that will be required in the run leg as much as possible on the bike leg.

CONCLUSION

Triathlon is a single sport consisting of three distinct, but connected, disciplines. As a result, training in one in the disciplines has to always be approached with the other two disciplines in mind.

Because the purpose of triathlon is to secure the best overall time, sometimes it is necessary to complete one of the earlier disciplines in a slightly slower time, with an eye on energy conservation, in order to be stronger towards the end of the race, and therefore post a better overall time.

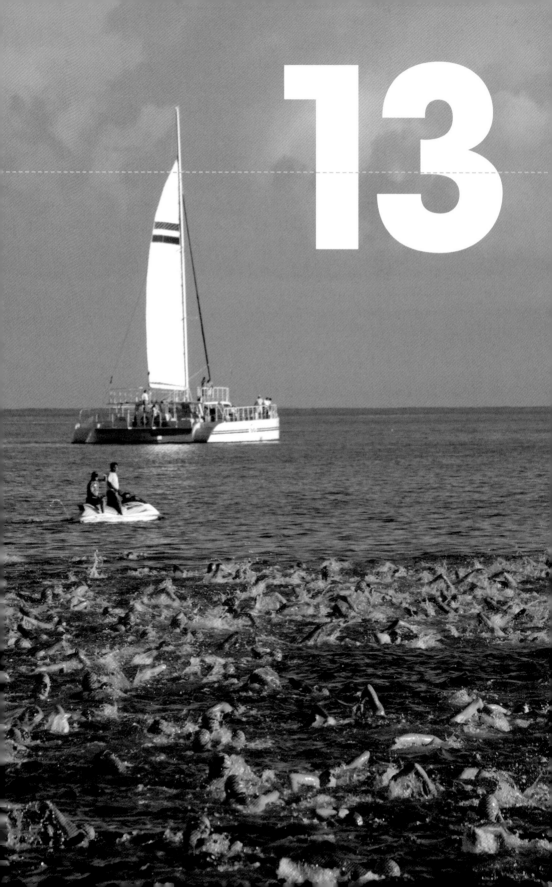

13

SWIMMING

The swimming discipline in triathlon is different from the other two disciplines in that, for the most part, it is a primarily upper body activity. As such, it requires specific training and different muscle use than regular single-sport swimming.

That said, no one is going to learn to swim properly with an efficient stroke by reading about it in a book. Swimming technique is all about doing it – good technique instruction and time spent in the water refining it. As a result, this chapter does not tell you how to swim. Instead, it provides some triathlon-specific swimming tips and advice on triathlon-specific subjects, such as open water swimming.

GET A SWIMMING COACH

As you step up your commitment to triathlon and implement that desire to move from a beginner to an intermediate-level masters triathlete, you need to employ the services of a good swimming coach to evaluate your stroke and give sound instruction on how to improve it and become more efficient.

A swimming coach is going to be additional to having a regular triathlon coach, unless you are fortunate enough to have a regular triathlon coach who is also a good swimming coach. Regular technical swimming instruction will benefit you just as much as endurance training sessions and increased time spent in the water.

In addition, joining a masters swim programme at the local swimming pool will add variety to your training, add an element of competitiveness, provide much-needed social interaction, and be a source of advice from both the resident session swimming coach and your fellow swimmers.

OPEN WATER SWIMMING

Three of the main facets unique to triathlon swimming over regular single-sport swimming are:

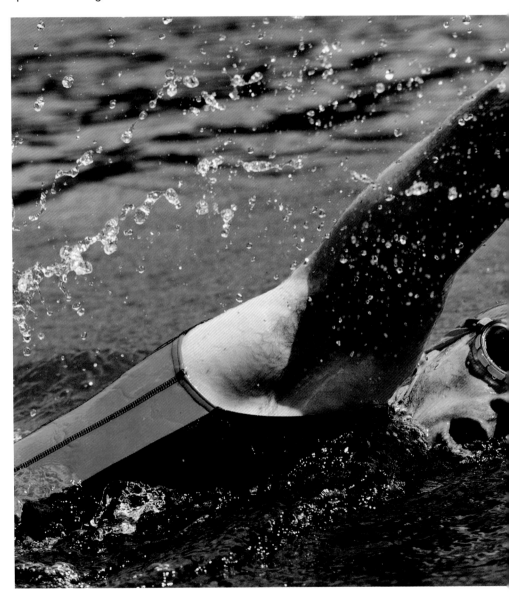

- getting comfortable swimming in open water;
- learning how to sight properly between the marker buoys and then swimming straight;
- learning how to draft off other swimmers.

As you step up from sprint distance triathlons to Olympic, half-Ironman and full Ironman distances, so you end up spending more time in open water during a race – up to 2 hours or more for an Ironman. Not only that, but that

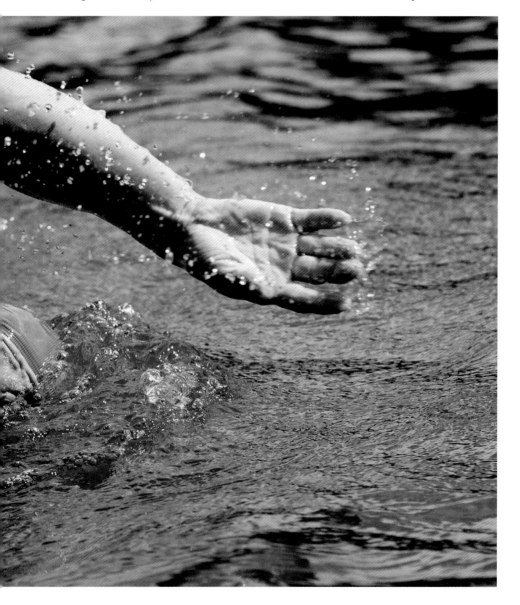

invariably means moving further away from the shoreline into deeper water – a psychological Grand Canyon!

Most people have, if not a fear of swimming in deep, open water, then at least nervousness about it. We have all at some point been culturally and psychologically affected (read damaged!) by the movie *Jaws*, and the immortal line, 'We're going to need a bigger boat.'

As a result, coupled with the need to increase swimming training volume is the need to become more comfortable with swimming in open water, with or without a wetsuit. How this is achieved depends on the upcoming season schedule.

There is no point practising swimming in a wetsuit if your two 'A' races for the season are both in warm water where wetsuits are not allowed, or training in the open ocean when you will be racing in small lakes or rivers. Training – both for swimming and for non-swimming – needs to be specific to your races. This emphasises the importance of setting out a season-long schedule, and even a two-season-long schedule.

Wetsuit use

A wetsuit needs to fit the person wearing it properly. It needs to be tight or it will act as a drag in the water, even if it does keep you warm. There will also be the need to tweak your technique slightly when swimming in a wetsuit. For example, because of the tight wetsuit around your shoulders, a high elbow recovery may unnecessarily fatigue your shoulders and take something out of your energy reserves.

One major benefit to swimming in a wetsuit, however, is that it keeps you buoyant with no additional energy expenditure on your part. As a result, the muscles and effort normally used to provide buoyancy – for example, keeping the hips and legs higher in the water so as not to act as a drag moving forward – can be saved for later in the race.

Anxiety

Anxiety, to a great extent, comes about because of lack of control. If you are in control of a situation, you are much less inclined to be anxious. The same mental technique that helps reduce anxiety in open water is the same mental technique that helps you stay motivated in training: focus only on those things that you can control.

When training in deep, open water, often with very limited visibility, you have to ignore the environmental elements that cannot be controlled, and focus only on those elements that you personally can control: regular swim technique, any additional open water swim technique, sighting and breathing. Block everything else out of your mind.

Hopefully, you will have done enough swimming in pools, and put in enough 'swim time', to have developed a 'feel' for the water, and to be comfortable at a certain pace and physical exertion. Subsequently, there is the need to focus on transferring that comfortable swimming pace that you have in the pool to the open water, both in training and in the race. Tense muscles mean extra exertion and laboured breathing. So relax and find your swimming comfort zone and apply it to the open water.

Sighting

Sighting – lifting the head to see where you are going – is a vital part of open water swimming. It becomes even more important in the open ocean or a large lake where even a little bit of chop can prevent you from seeing the course buoys and possibly send you off in the wrong direction. No one wants to swim further than necessary.

However, the key to sighting is to lift the head as little as possible. Think of the body as being like a seesaw with the fulcrum right around where the hips are. Lift the head up even a little and the feet drop down, adding to drag in the water. As a result, the head should only be lifted as high as is needed to sight, and no more.

The best triathletes sight in a smooth, fluid action, at the same time as taking a breath to the side in their normal breathing sequence, either before or after the breath. The head comes up to the side to take a breath, and in the same movement it circles around to the front to snatch a quick glance forward to see where the next buoy is located. The act of sighting should not interrupt the rhythm of the swim stroke or add to the drag of the body and make it more inefficient in the water.

Even though most beach-based swimming starts will have the first leg of the swim travelling away from shore, and therefore often with no land behind the first turn buoy, subsequent buoys on the swim course may have land somewhere behind them, in the distance. The result is that you can often sight something higher on land behind the buoy, rather than the ocean-level buoy itself, which will often be obscured by choppy water.

If it is not possible to scout the swim course the day before the race, be sure to give yourself enough time at the start to identify possible landmarks that can be used while swimming.

Drafting

Just like the cycling legs in draft-legal triathlons such as those governed by the International Triathlon Union, drafting in the swimming leg of any triathlon (i.e. swimming directly behind, or behind and to the side, of a fellow competitor) can save 20 to 25 per cent on expended energy. Particularly with the longer half-Ironman and full Ironman distances, that is a lot of saved energy you will definitely be thankful for later in the race. In addition, drafting behind someone faster than you can improve your overall time. Drafting just behind someone, almost touching their toes, is the conventional way of drafting, but

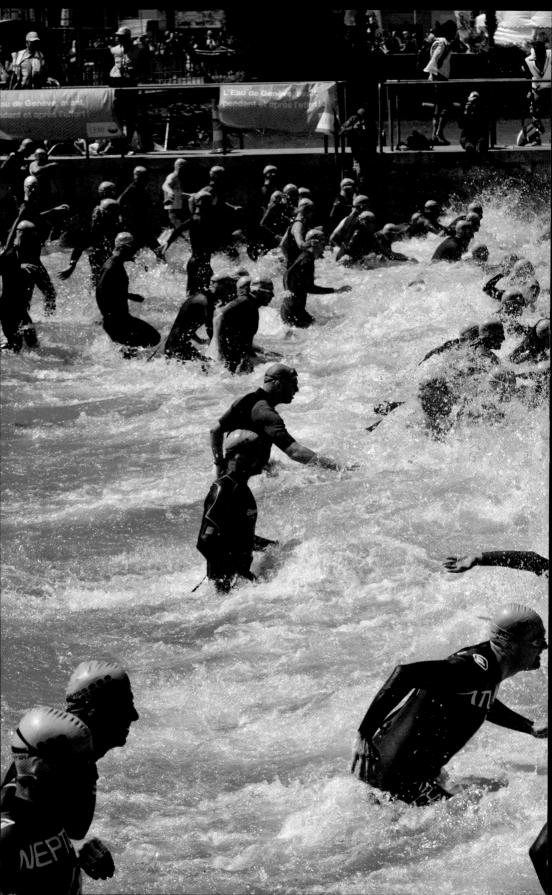

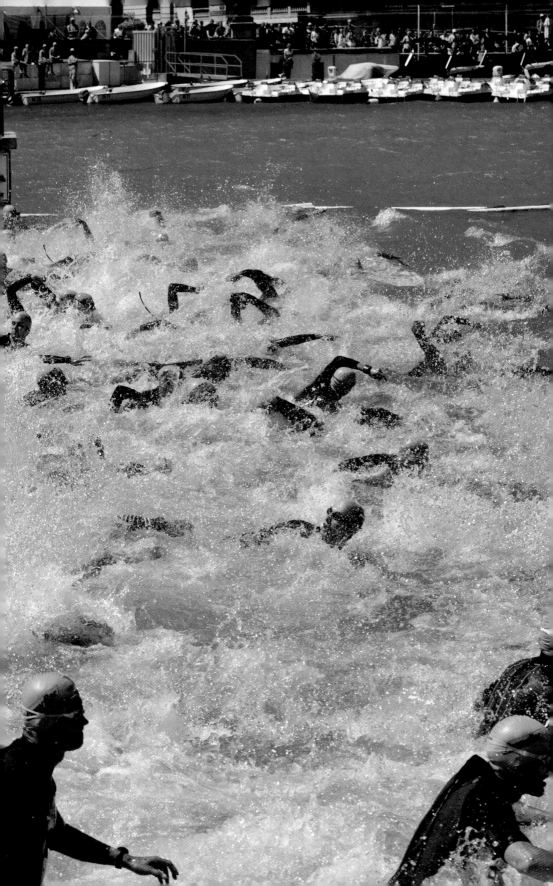

be careful not to touch them or interfere with their rhythm. Drafting close to the side of someone, so your head is between their chest and hips, allows your body to swim in the wake they generate, just like with a motor boat.

Both drafting techniques take practice to execute effectively without impeding the other swimmer. Practising the technique in the pool or in open water with a training partner before a race will pay dividends.

SWIMMING TECHNIQUE TIPS

- Many fundamental improvements in technique involve the placement of the head and the notion that the body is a kind of seesaw with the fulcrum around the hips. Lift the front end of the seesaw and the back end goes down. If the back end goes down, it adds to drag in the water and will slow the swimmer down.

- Keep the head face down in the water, looking directly below you. Keep the head and body in a straight line, like a wooden board. Only lift the head up and forward on the sighting stroke. On a breathing stroke, the idea is not to lift the head out of the water but to roll the head to the side just enough for your mouth to clear the water and be able to take a breath, and no more.

- Another tip also involves the seesaw effect. In swimming it is called 'pressing your buoy'. This notion seems to go in and out of fashion, but putting it into practice to some degree makes sense. The lungs are like balloons, filled with air. As a result, they are more likely to rise to the surface than sink. Using the seesaw effect, if you can push down slightly with your head and chest in the water as you swim, your legs will rise slightly towards the surface. This makes it less necessary to kick the legs to raise the butt and legs up and streamline the body in a straight line, therefore conserving energy for the rest of the triathlon.

- The legs and lower body are not really there for propulsion. You have to preserve their muscles as best you can for the two leg-based disciplines that follow. Conserve as much energy as possible by having the legs relaxed in the water, kicking in a slow, rhythmical fashion. Many middle- and long-distance triathlon swimmers choose to kick in unison with their stroke. This synchronises all the limbs together, creating a smooth, overall fluid rhythm that conserves energy.

- Swim with a high elbow under the water when executing the arm pull, allowing the hand to come closer to the chest with the forearm facing backwards rather than down, thus reducing drag from having a straight arm, while at the same time increasing efficiency and propulsion.

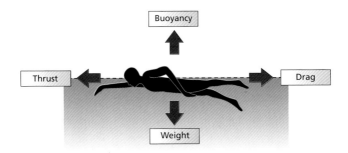

Factors that impact swimming

TECHNIQUE TIPS

Unless you are coming from a swimming background, a triathlete, even one that spends 20 hours training for the sport every week, is unlikely to be at the same level as a good swimmer who has been focusing on only swimming training for years. It is simply a question of time in the water. In triathlon, there are three disciplines to focus on, plus gym and strength work. With a single discipline, you have just that: a single discipline to spend all your time on.

With swimming, technique is everything. Good technique means efficiency. Efficiency in the water means speed, with less energy expended. As a result, the importance of constant swim instruction and technique evaluation is paramount. However, with so many moving parts to pay attention to, it can often be overwhelming for someone trying to move up from the beginner level to the intermediate level to know what to focus on first.

The box opposite shows five key technique pointers to focus on initially in order to improve efficiency and speed.

CONCLUSION

Of the three triathlon disciplines, swimming is the one that benefits most from good technique, but suffers most from bad technique. The result is that personal technique instruction is not only recommended, it is a 'must'. So find a good swimming coach, and listen to what they say!

In addition, swim stroke and speed will improve with practice time spent in the water. However, extra care should be taken by masters swimmers to avoid repetitive injuries to both the shoulders and the elbows. Better technique means more efficiency and less energy used, but it also means less stress on the muscles and joints, as increased efficiency also means less resistance in the water and less stress on the body as a result.

1894

14

CYCLING

The longest part of any triathlon race, and any triathlon training schedule, will be spent on the bike. A weak bike leg, or over-exertion on the bike leg, will not only take you back down the field, but will often result in a failure to finish the run section altogether.

This book is not intended to provide instruction on how to ride a bike. Instead, this chapter offers a few pointers that can be focused on to improve triathlon cycling – from cycling position to pedal stroke, to the importance of bike handling skills – in the move from beginner to intermediate triathlete.

CYCLING POSITION ON THE BIKE

In cycling, an estimated 80 per cent of the wind resistance is caused by the rider and 20 per cent by the bike. In addition, wind resistance accounts for as much as 85 per cent of the resistance that needs to be overcome. As a result, the rider's cycling position becomes paramount.

Cycling position is initially more important than aerodynamic equipment such as wheels and helmet. Having aerodynamic equipment is irrelevant if the riding position itself is so non-aerodynamic that it is contributing to increased resistance.

For anyone wanting to get faster on the bike, the first step is to have their riding position checked by a professional to make sure the riding angles are all correct in relation to the handlebars, saddle and pedals. So make an appointment at a local bike shop that offers that service.

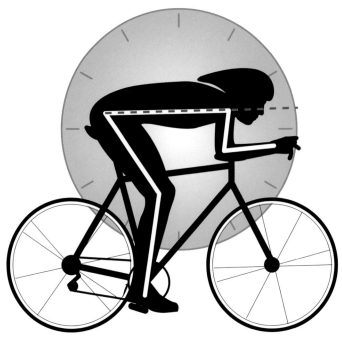

Optimum triathlon bike body position

CIRCULAR PEDALLING

Most beginner-level cyclists, and probably too many intermediate-level cyclists, pedal by simply pushing down on the downward part of the pedal stroke and do not pay enough attention to pulling up through the second part of the action as the stroke goes through its full rotation of 360°. However, cycling in a down–up circular motion helps generate a higher power output by engaging more muscles.

It is important to control the pedal stroke and not let the pedal stroke control you. You need to be in control of the full 360° rotation of the pedal stroke and not have any dead spots where the pedals and chain seem to slip and feel disengaged. Pedal stroke can be practised using both single leg drills and double leg drills to ensure correct circular rotation.

PROPER FORM

Coupled with a circular pedalling technique, rather than an incomplete press-down technique, correct cycling form will help in training, build up cycling strength in all the right areas of the body and help prevent injuries by making cycling muscles stronger.

One aspect of correct cycling form is to keep the trunk and body as still as possible while pedalling. Too much side-to-side and up-and-down motion in the trunk and body adds to inefficiency and bad aerodynamics.

Much of the power for cycling comes from the quads, thighs and gluteus maximus muscles. You should be able to sustain a comfortable race pace just using those muscle groups as a driver. If you find yourself struggling to stay still because you are grinding out a hard gear, it is time to change to a slightly easier, more fluid gear that allows the body to remain stable.

Of the three disciplines, cycling is the one that requires the least work from the upper body. As a result, relaxing the upper body on the ride, while keeping it as stable as possible, will make it become more efficient and aerodynamic. In addition, keeping a relaxed upper body will use up less valuable oxygen that can then be used for energy generation in the legs and glute muscle groups.

CADENCE

There is an ongoing debate about cadence in triathlon cycling. That is because triathlon cycling is not 'single-sport' cycling. With triathlon cycling, you still have the run afterwards, which is inevitably performed with tired leg muscles.

The easiest way to calculate pedal stroke revolutions per minute on the fly is to count the number of times the right foot completes a 360° pedal rotation in 10 seconds and multiply that number by six.

With regular cycling, a high cadence of 80–100 revolutions per minute is regarded favourably because it allows the rider to maintain fast speeds with less stress on the leg muscles, and is often seen as the optimum way to generate pedal power.

There is a school of thought, however, that advocates the use of bigger gears in triathlon cycling, with a lower cadence whenever possible, in order to preserve the fast-twitch muscle fibres for the fatigue-shortened run stride of the run. Such a technique also keeps the heart rate low on the bike, which in turn allows for the use of fat in the generation of energy and not the more valuable (and limited) carbohydrates, which will be used for the run. Higher cadence on the bike, so the argument goes, means greater aerobic effort, which means you are more likely to use carbohydrates than fat for energy.

Whatever cadence you use throughout the bike section of the triathlon, everyone is faced with the same problem at the end: the actual physical transition from cycling to running. There are different muscle demands in cycling to those on the run. The best triathletes cope with those changes seemingly effortlessly. The reality though, is that they practise hard in their training for the physiological changes those two disciplines demand.

One tip that every calibre of triathlete can adopt is to increase the cadence on the bike in the last mile or so of the bike leg, while changing into an easier gear. This allows the muscles in the legs to get a head start and adjust to the different physiological demands when they transition from bike pedalling to the fast leg turnover of a run.

PROPER SHIFTING

Whatever cadence and gear selection you decide to go with, it is important to maintain it without speeding up and slowing down uncontrollably, for example, in response to the terrain. Which is why bikes have gears! Proper shifting to maintain a steady cadence and a given gear selection, in order to conserve energy and lower the heart rate, is imperative.

Proper gear selection takes practice, and coordination with a heart rate monitor, cycling computer, and whatever sensory techniques you have developed in unison with your coach. Incorrect shifting will create unnecessary fatigue, deplete vital carbohydrate stores and use valuable energy that will be required for the run.

BREATHING

Breathing in any endurance sport is all about rhythm, and triathlon cycling is no different. Simply put, your breathing should be rhythmically synchronised with your pedal stroke. Even a sprint triathlon will have a comparatively long time in the saddle.

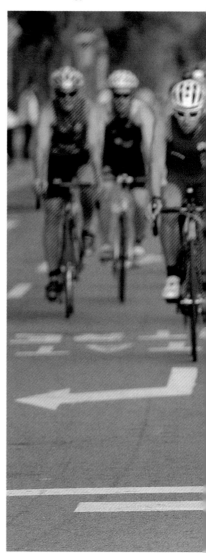

As a result, breathing should always be under control. The more control you have of your breathing, the more control you have over your heart rate, which means the more efficient you will be in producing energy to power your muscles.

In addition, as mentioned previously, keeping your breathing controlled and your heart rate low will allow you to burn fat for energy and not have to resort to the more valuable carbohydrates.

DON'T TAX THE RUN MUSCLES

It has been mentioned already about the importance of cycling in a way that taxes the run muscles and depletes valuable carbohydrates as little as possible. It is worth mentioning again though. Wherever possible, it makes sense to ride at a low cadence, but in a bigger gear, while maintaining the same race speed, because at that rate the body will utilise fat in the production of energy (which powers the muscles) rather than the more valuable carbohydrates.

Running raises the heart rate and oxygen consumption very quickly compared to cycling.

As the heart rate goes up at the outset of the run, and breathing becomes laboured, the body at some point will switch to carbohydrates instead of fat to produce energy, except that fat supplies are far more abundant in a body than carbohydrates. So ride in a way that suits you, but does not unnecessarily tax the run muscles and deplete the vital energy supplies that will be used on the run later.

RACE-SPECIFIC TRAINING

Even though there are certain bike handling skills that need to be practised no matter what your race schedule for the season looks like – for example,

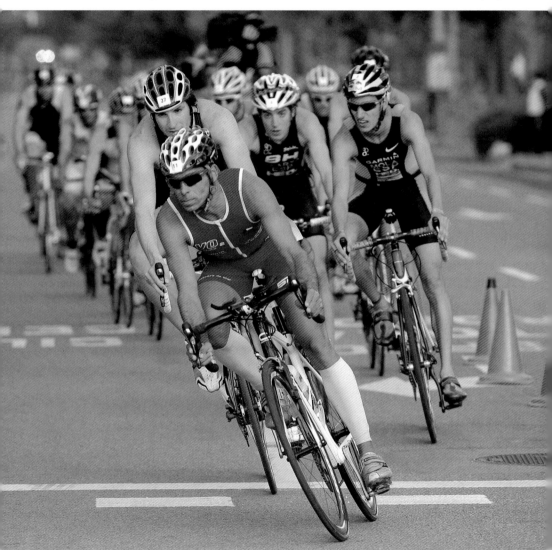

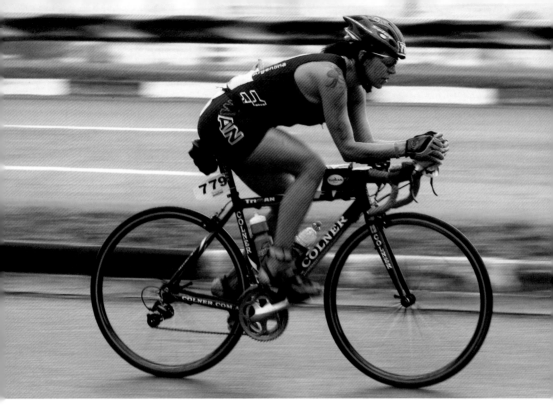

descending and cornering – one of the values of a season-long triathlon plan is that it allows you to focus your training on the skills you will require in the upcoming race.

For example, if you are going to tackle a tough and hilly Ironman course in 4 months' time, there is little value in always training on flat, aerobar-friendly rides. Of course, you have to include that type of training in your schedule, but if the race is a long, hilly course, you should be focusing on long, hilly training rides.

Once you have completed one race, you should then adapt your training to the next 'A' race in the season. Having 2–4 months between 'A' races allows you to virtually start again after each race with a specific training schedule focused on the upcoming race and the type of terrain and environmental conditions you will face. Just as one size does not fit all for the personal training schedules of triathletes, so one size does not fit all when it comes to race-specific training schedules.

BIKE HANDLING SKILLS

If you participate in a triathlon race where there are many hundreds of other competitors in close proximity, the least you can do is make sure you are not endangering any of them by inadequate bike skills. If your lack of bike handling skills causes an accident at 15–20 miles per hour, or even slower, the result is very likely to be broken bones for someone.

One way to practise close-quarters bike handling skills is the same way you would practise car handling skills at low speeds: place some cones close together in an empty parking lot and ride slowly around them, decreasing the distance between the cones, and speeding up as your handling skills increase.

Once you have acquired rudimentary bike handling skills, join a group ride for some of your training rides. Aside from getting comfortable with riding in close proximity to others, even though there are few triathlon races for age-groupers that allow draft-legal group riding on the course, a group ride also gives you a social outlet in what is for the most part a very solitary sport for training.

In addition, try to ride with people who are better than you are, at least occasionally. No one ever really gets better, or realises their full potential, by only riding with people that are the same level as them, or even at a lower level. Riding with people who are better than you are makes you step up your game to stay with them. It will also teach you the art of drafting in a hurry whether you will need it in a race or not!

No matter what your upcoming races for the season, you need to practise your descending skills, and especially your cornering skills. Even if you plan on only participating in 'flat' races, you will be doing a lot of climbing and descending in training, and even more cornering, sometimes at considerable speeds. You can make up a lot of time on descents, which can kill two valuable birds with one stone: provide you with much-needed recovery when you do not need to pedal, while at the same time making up overall time with better descending skills than your competitors.

CONCLUSION

Proficiency in cycling definitely does not come overnight with regard to both fitness and bike handling skills. Moving up from beginner to intermediate in cycling inevitably entails a huge jump in fitness, but also increased danger as greater sustained speeds are attained and longer time is spent training on the road. Injury prevention in triathlon is of paramount concern, and in the case of cycling this applies to accident prevention too.

Better cycling technique will lead to better performance with little extra aerobic effort on the part of the rider. Cycling looks straightforward, but it is the small technical aspects – pedal stroke and body positioning on the bike, for example – that will help a triathlete make that step up to the next level.

Additionally, because of the amount of time spent on the bike in any distance triathlon race, it is the cycling section where most time gains, at least initially, will be made as cycling proficiency improves.

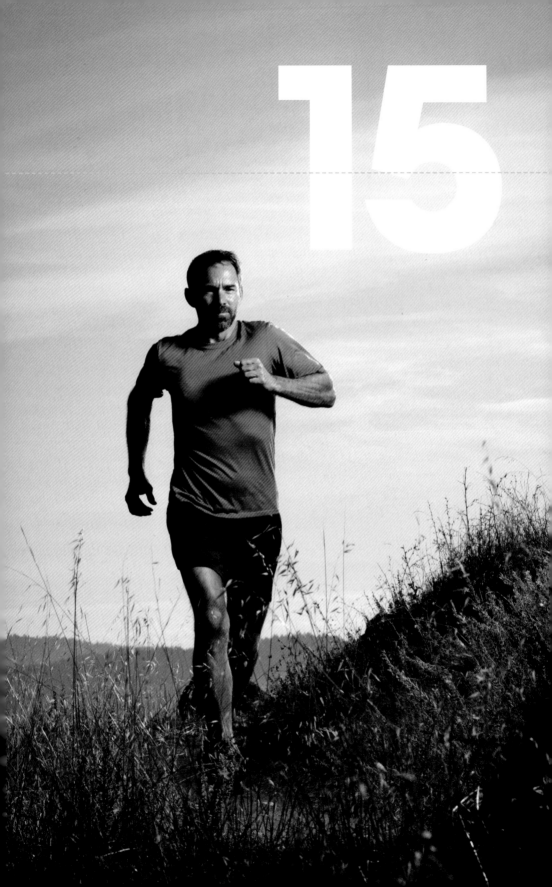

15

RUNNING

**THREE MASTERS CONSIDERATIONS
DISCUSSED IN THIS CHAPTER:**

- In addition to regularly buying new running shoes in an effort to prevent impact injuries, masters athletes should run on softer ground, such as grass, whenever possible.

- Correct running technique will save energy by being more efficient.

- The older you get, the more important it is to lose the 'junk' miles and focus each run workout on quality rather than quantity.

There is an old saying in triathlon that 'The bike is for show, but the run is for the dough.' The bottom line for all triathletes is that, no matter how good you are at cycling or swimming, you still have to complete the run. And if you want to be on the podium, you have to complete it fast. The run is where the race is won or lost, where personal bests are mainly improved, and where most DNFs occur.

This chapter is not about running fundamentals, but about running-related issues for triathletes, and in particular masters triathletes. Some of these issues are controversial, including stride length and high-intensity workouts.

RUNNING IS RUNNING?

Running is running, whether it is a stand-alone sport or one of three disciplines within the sport of triathlon, right? Actually, the answer is no.

While the basic mechanics of athletic running remain the same, many would argue there is a different focus for triathlon running that does not exist with stand-alone running. That focus has to do with the two disciplines that come before the run on a triathlon.

The key to a successful triathlon is efficiency and energy conservation in an effort to maximise total race time over all three disciplines, not just how fast you can perform one of the three disciplines. Often that entails going slower than you would normally go in the swim and/or the cycling in order to conserve energy for the discipline that follows. It can also involve changing how you execute technique in order to maximise deteriorating energy and physiological resources towards the end of the race.

The case in point here is running. Of course, there is an optimal running technique that will maximise efficiency and speed in order to complete an endurance run in the fastest possible time. The problem with a triathlon is that when the run discipline actually begins, a triathlete's leg muscles are already fatigued to some degree from the cycling stage.

As a result, the cycling portion of the race should be completed in such a way that minimises fatigue to the run muscles. A balance has to be reached between aerobic and cycling fatigue from the bike, and starting the run with the running muscles as fresh as possible, with enough left in them to complete the race without dramatic athletic decline.

Triathlon is all about balance and maximising the declining physical resources that you have at your disposal. While a stand-alone cycling race may involve considerable amounts of fast-cadence cycling using slightly easier gears in an effort to create power, that method comes at an increased aerobic price for a triathlete, because it will eat into the glycogen reserves that really need to be saved for the triathlon run. Not only that, but a faster cadence requires use of fast-twitch muscle fibres. Why is that important?

One school of triathlon thought argues that, because you reach the start of the run in a highly fatigued state, it will not be long before your run technique inevitably begins to suffer as a result. When that happens, run muscles will fatigue, you range of motion will decline due to overused and tight muscles, muscles will cramp, and stride length will shorten as a result. This is especially true with the longer distances rather than the short sprint and even Olympic-distance races. When that happens, if you maintain the same run cadence as you did when you started the run, you will inevitably slow down.

The most obvious remedy is to shorten stride length and increase cadence in order to compensate, and therefore maintain your overall pace.

However, increasing run cadence and shortening stride length is an acquired expertise that needs to be addressed in training. Just as for the bike, increasing run cadence also increases aerobic demand. Unlike the bike, however, raising the heart rate as a result of increasing run cadence happens very quickly, placing immediate increased demand on the ever-dwindling stores of glycogen. In addition, increased cadence and shortened stride length requires the firing of the all-important fast-twitch muscle fibres, which decline with age.

The importance of a cycling technique that keeps heart rate down – such as using a bigger chain ring that requires more leg muscle strength rather than increased aerobic demand (which in turn allows for the use of fat as a source of energy because the heart rate is lower, and not carbohydrates and glycogen) – is evident. Such a cycling technique also makes less of a demand

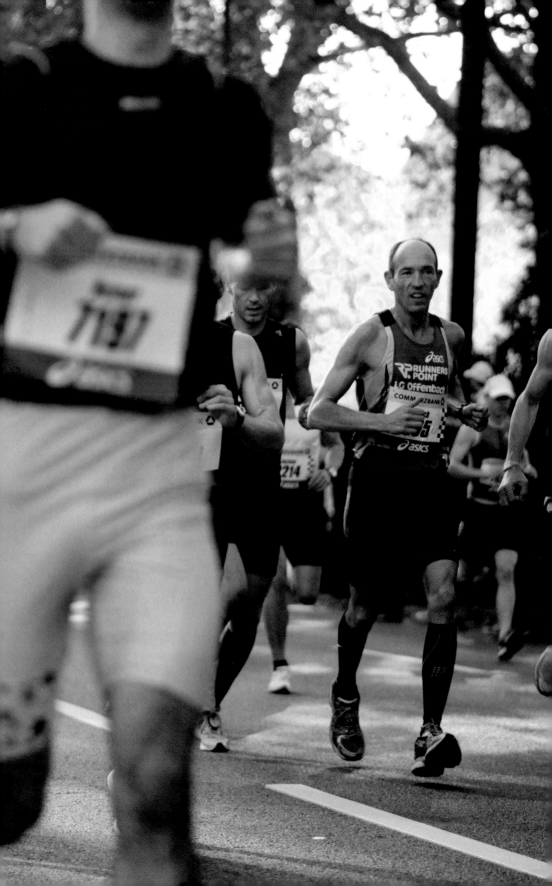

on the fast-twitch muscle fibres that will be required on the run because of the resulting shortened stride length and increased run cadence.

One argument says to increase efficiency in endurance triathlon running by adopting a higher cadence with a shortened stride length. The longer the triathlon run, such as with Ironman or half-Ironman distances, the greater the importance in adopting such a style. Muscle fatigue and tightness, as well as cramping, necessitates such a change, but it can only be implemented effectively over a long distance if the technique is practised in training.

It is widely known that, while strength and power can wane quickly with age, endurance for a fit athlete barely declines at all. One often-quoted figure is that a fit athlete will only lose 4 per cent of their endurance by the time they are 55.

Indeed, training with the same ongoing intensity as you enter masters age groups often results in very little athletic decline. Maintaining a similar training intensity slows performance decline and can sustain a competitive body well into the sixties and seventies.

TRAINING CHANGES AS YOU AGE

That said, there are some changes that need to be made to a training regimen as the body ages.

The first changes in run training involve focus and frequency. The youthful days of long, 'junk' mileage need to be phased out. It is no longer quantity that is required for the masters runner, but quality. Every workout should be a quality workout, pre-planned with session goals and targets.

However, cutting back on training volume need not be the result. Indeed, there have been numerous examples of athletes who have increased their volume with age, with positive results, especially if they did little volume in their younger days.

In addition, as with all masters workouts, training should be carried out with one eye on injury prevention. As a result, run training days should have a non-run day in between – perhaps totalling no more than two or three run training days a week. High-intensity run workouts should ideally have a rest day after. Also, not all run days will be at a high intensity.

This being triathlon, with three disciplines requiring regular training and enough hours, you might have to settle for a swim the day following a run coupled with a ride, or a swim coupled with strength training for the upper body and non-run muscles, instead of a rest day.

Strength training, especially for the upper body, is as important for running as it is for swimming. In addition, strength training helps with weight management in all masters athletes, not just those who consider themselves overweight.

As the body ages, it goes thorough physiological changes, which include an increase in fat, especially in the upper body, as well as a decrease in muscle mass. Resistance training and lifting weights helps keep fat at bay, along with slowing down the decline in muscle mass and bone density.

HIGH-INTENSITY AND WELL-PLANNED WORKOUTS

High-intensity workouts become more difficult because of certain physiological developments: fat contributes to a narrowing of the blood vessels, the heart's walls stiffen, and cardiac strength declines.

As a result, workouts that feature interval runs with short recoveries maintain a high oxygen consumption, which helps increase VO_2 max, as well as increasing fast-twitch muscle fibres. High-intensity workouts are essential to maintaining aerobic capacity.

Maintaining intensity for masters athletes as they age, and even including more high-intensity run workouts, is an important part of maintaining high-level competitive and athletic capabilities.

Cutting back on training time, certainly without an increase in quality in the workouts, is a sure way to lose fitness in masters athletes. By contrast, high mileage and the lack of complete recovery days is the primary cause of injury in older runners. As the body becomes more prone to injury, especially related to running, athletes should consider cutting down high mileage in favour of high-quality, high-intensity workouts.

Adding an extra recovery day during the training week, along with lowering mileage, can go a long way to preventing injury. Meanwhile, high-intensity workouts improve VO_2 max decline, often resulting in the posting of better personal run times. The extra recovery day from the leg- and knee-pounding of run training and the added focus and pre-planning of higher-quality workouts can also result in less tissue damage.

In addition, with the possible reduction of long mileage-focused training and the transition to more focused, better-planned and higher-intensity run workouts, hard sessions should also begin to be more race-specific.

While there is overlap in all run training for masters athletes, especially if you include high-intensity workouts in the training week as a matter of course, there comes a point where there is little to be gained with general run training, and much to be lost with the overexposure to possible injury. Training with an emphasis on half-marathon-oriented mileage, for example, if you are only planning sprint triathlon 5K runs for the coming season, makes no sense.

That said, any running speed work needs to be approached with caution for the masters athlete because of the way muscles and related connective tissues lose their elasticity and flexibility as the body ages. Introducing yoga as a way to combat such declines or exposure to speed-related strains, in place of a third or fourth run workout each week, can bear fruit in the long term.

Speed work is most likely to be high in intensity, but not all high-intensity training is necessarily speed work. If the intended races do not call for speed work, then masters athletes should seriously consider cutting back on it for the most part. Fast-twitch muscle fibres, for example, can be stimulated by training other than speed work.

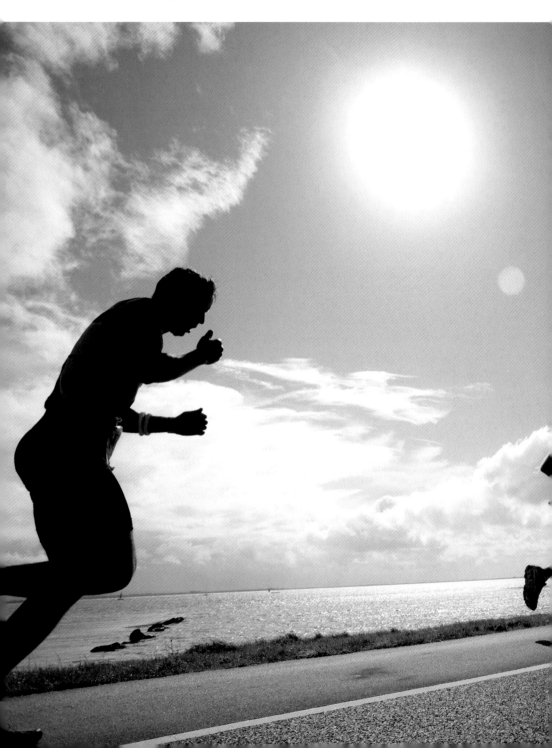

CONCLUSION

Because running is the hardest of all three triathlon disciplines on the muscles, connective tissues and joints, it is the one where most care is needed in training to prevent injury and damage, especially in masters athletes. For the most part, a more focused, race-specific and often higher-intensity approach to running training for masters athletes as they age is preferable to the continuous pounding of long runs, even though low-intensity, high-volume runs do inevitably still have their place if you are training for the longer triathlons such as Ironman and half-Ironman distances.

A more balanced, well-planned training approach for running that includes high-intensity workouts will benefit the masters body most, and not just in regard to triathlon, but in health generally.

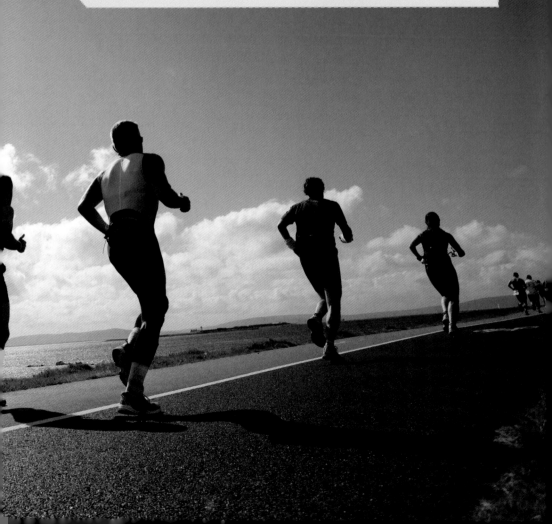

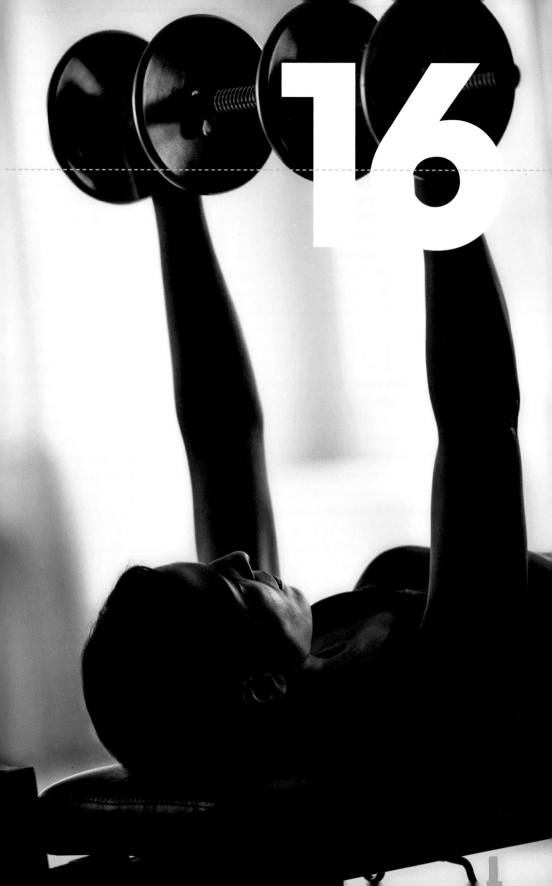

16

STRENGTH TRAINING

**THREE MASTERS CONSIDERATIONS
DISCUSSED IN THIS CHAPTER:**

- Strength training is vital because of the body's normal age-related muscle mass decline.

- It is vital to recognise the difference between exercise-induced muscle soreness and possible injury, because muscles tend to hurt more with age.

- Strength training aids good technique, which in turn allows an athlete to be more efficient for longer.

Just as good technique is essential in triathlon, so is muscle strength. Gym work and weight training are a crucial part of any triathlon training programme, especially for masters athletes, and should be in everyone's ongoing weekly training schedule.

For masters athletes, the losses of muscle mass and bone density, as well as muscle strength, are some of the most pronounced effects of aging, although those losses can vary with age and the actual muscle groups involved. Nevertheless, some sources put the actual muscle mass loss at as much as 15 per cent per decade for someone in their sixties or seventies, and as much as 30 per cent in those older.

STRENGTH TRAINING PREVENTS MUSCLE MASS DECLINE

The main casualty of all this muscle loss is the fast-twitch muscle fibres that provide, for example, explosive power and reaction time. However, muscle mass decline can be slowed down by high-intensity training, in endurance and sprint workouts, and in power and strength training. As a result, weight training for masters athletes is critical, from a triathlon perspective, but also from the perspective of quality of life and general motor skills.

While the off-season is likely to be the best place in a yearly training schedule for a greater volume of strength training – always supervised and within safe limits – it is necessary to include weight and strength training year-round to maintain muscular strength. How much depends on an athlete's personal considerations, training schedule and timetable.

Strength training also helps keep the heart strong. The heart, having reached its peak condition in an athlete's twenties and thirties, will begin to lose power and efficiency over time. A fit athlete's maximum heart capacity will also decline. The most often-quoted rule of thumb for calculating maximum heart rate is to subtract your age from 220 for men, and from 226 for women. Everyone is different, of course, because of genetics and fitness, among other considerations. As a result, heart capacity can vary between two triathletes of similar build and athletic abilities.

Training at a maximum heart rate is not possible for very long. Much of a triathlete's target training rate will be about 80 per cent of maximum heart rate.

There are two primary reasons that strength training is essential to masters athletes. The first, as already mentioned, is that it helps maintain both declining muscle mass and declining bone mass. Fast-twitch muscle can never be fully replaced as the body ages, but strength training can go a long way to filling the void.

The second reason is that it requires strength to maintain good technique once the body begins to tire. Good technique increases efficiency, which not only makes you go faster for longer, but also helps to prevent injuries. Once good technique falls by the wayside, dangerous stresses and strains are placed on muscles and joints to maintain speed. As the body gets even more fatigued, those stresses and strains become more pronounced, leading to injuries.

There are a number of additional reasons for weight and strength training for a masters athlete. Resistance training can enhance muscle mass and function, as well as add to muscular power in masters athletes, and is particularly effective in athletes over 70. High-velocity resistance training in older athletes, particularly as it relates to the large muscle groups such as the thighs, can prevent significant reduced power declines, and indeed sometimes lead to power improvements.

There are considerable general health benefits for older people from strength training, whether they are athletes or not. Aside from helping combat the aforementioned muscle mass decline, it can help normalise high blood pressure, improve posture and help with weight control by increasing the resting metabolic rate post-workout, and therefore reducing body fat.

It can also help treat and even prevent osteoporosis – a major problem for older women – by increasing bone density and therefore bone strength, and as a result reduce pain as well as improving function. There is also medical evidence that demonstrates it can help type 2 diabetes sufferers by reducing their resistance to insulin.

Additionally, it can also reduce stress (as exercise generally can), and increase quality of life in older people by reducing the risk of falls, which is the primary cause of injuries to the aged.

From an athletic perspective, strength-training increases fast-twitch muscle fibres, which are necessary for explosive reaction time, power generation and speed.

Running efficiency is tied to muscle strength. Unlike swimming, which is virtually a non-weight-bearing discipline, the muscles in running must be strong enough to support the load-bearing running action of the lower body over long and fatigue-inducing distances. However, while with swimming efficient technique trumps brute strength every time, because of the benefits that efficiency and smooth technique contribute towards speed in the water, the load-bearing nature of running requires muscle strength to maintain motion efficiency.

Increased muscle strength also means reduced energy consumption, which is vital for the run segment in a triathlon, because fewer muscles are needed to support the same load and effort. The load in running is going to remain the same, whatever the triathletes' muscle strength. So the stronger the muscles involved relative to the demands of the exercise, and therefore the fewer muscles required, the better.

Increased muscle also allows for the use of more oxygen, which improves endurance performance. Strength training has been shown to increase the lactate threshold in athletes, which is vital to endurance athletes. Interestingly, some research also shows that, to an extent, a certain amount of endurance training can be replaced by strength training without there being a loss of endurance fitness.

In association with the ability to sustain correct technique and prevent dangerous stresses and strains on the joints and muscles as fatigue sets in, strength training also contributes to more stable joints by strengthening the connective tissues.

Increased muscle strength also helps improve athlete confidence and mental positivity, which is a huge part of success in triathlon.

PROGRAMME CONSIDERATIONS

The same initial considerations that apply to the separate disciplines of swimming, cycling and running also apply to a strength development programme. Without wishing to sound like a broken record, everyone is different, so at the outset it may take half a dozen workout sessions to determine a triathlete's workload, weights, repetitions and general fitness with regard to weight and strength training.

The same adage applies to strength training as for other triathlon training: start slow and light, with plenty of recovery, and build up from there.

For the masters athlete, the age-specific considerations also add to the need for caution. This can include an already declined muscle mass, with a resulting strength and power reduction from younger years and the need for additional recovery to give muscles time to strengthen and grow. It can also involve a more variable and volatile mental approach that can run the gamut from believing they can do more than their body is capable of to a belief that their body is beyond gaining any benefit from weight training, resulting in a lack of motivation and effort.

The bottom line is that, for any older athlete, the rules of adaptation still apply. With age, though, more variables come into play, or at least variables with greater consequences. With adaptation, subject the muscles to stresses and break the muscles down, then add recovery time to give those muscles enough time to rebuild and come back stronger.

In a way, masters triathletes should be treated in the same way as those new to weight and strength training programmes. Even masters athletes accustomed to using weights in the gym, however intermittent their use, need to contend with the natural decline of muscle mass, as well as the resulting strength and power loss as the body ages.

As a result, any new strength programme (which also applies to the initial stages of any year-round programme) should start with lighter weights, few repetitions, a limited number of exercises and extended recovery periods in-between workouts. Masters athletes, when increasing intensity in strength training, should be wary of focusing on heavier weights with shorter repetitions, a common practice in weight training for younger athletes. Instead, the programme should include lighter weights with more repetitions.

In addition, correct technique is vital no matter the age of the athlete, and correct instruction for the exercise in question should be a fundamental initial part of any strength programme.

Physiological changes in athletes that come with age mean that what may have worked just a couple of years before in terms of technique and programme substance may not work now, or, worse, may actually be placing dangerous stresses on the joints and muscles.

It is natural for joints and muscles to hurt more for those athletes over 50 years of age following a workout. The key is to be able to distinguish between what is natural workout fatigue and what is abnormal pain caused by the onset of potential injury. As a result, constant supervision of any weight or strength programme is essential for masters athletes.

Continued pain and fatigue in the joints and muscles, even after what should be sufficient recovery time, will be likely to mean a backing off from the strength training and a possible medical visit to ensure no long-term damage or physiological abnormalities.

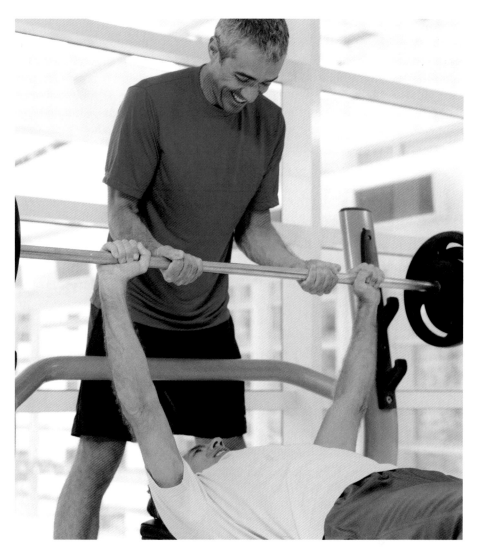

In addition, because of the natural decline of strength in the heart due to aging, any adverse effects of a strength programme, such as dizziness or nausea, should be taken seriously. High-intensity resistance training requires increased blood flow. Any health issue that could be the result of strength training and the resulting increased blood flow should be investigated with a qualified physician.

Also, as a precaution, masters athletes should be discouraged from lifting weights to complete failure, as well as holding their breath completely when lifting heavier weights, as this can raise blood pressure.

Strength training programmes should reduce intensity as age increases. Of particular importance, especially as bodies age in inconsistent physiological ways, is to use strength programmes to address and help correct any muscular inconsistencies.

Periodisation of strength training plans is as important as periodisation for general triathlon training schedules. As mentioned, extended recovery periods for both are essential because the body requires more time to rebuild as age increases. As a result, some triathlon-oriented strength approaches seek to mimic the periodisation progressions of regular triathlon training plans.

Strength exercises should be emphasised that replicate how the body, muscles and joints are used in the three disciplines – swimming, cycling and running – and triathlon demands generally.

Strength exercises that use multiple joints instead of single joints are usually preferable, because that is the way the body will be used in triathlon. Rarely are single joints used in triathlon in isolation. Wherever possible training should replicate race stresses.

FIVE STAGES OF PERIODISED STRENGTH TRAINING

There are five general stages of a triathlon-specific, periodised, strength programme. However, this being triathlon, that figure varies between coaches and training schedule approaches. So there could be seven, or there could be three! In addition, the different phases usually overlap. However, whether you have three or five stages in your strength programme, they will probably include these elements somewhere within the box below:

- **The base stage** of any strength programme prepares the body, muscles, tendons and joints for the heavy training workloads that will follow. Additionally, the focus of this initial stage is on general body strength. This is usually in the triathlon off-season over the winter where general triathlon training is at a minimum.

- **The endurance stage** targets the endurance-oriented slow-twitch muscle fibres that accompany any general aerobic-based triathlon schedule. This often accompanies the stage in a general triathlon training schedule where low-intensity, high-volume aerobic rides are the norm. Emphasis is also placed on coping with high lactate levels as endurance mileage increases.

- **The strength and power stage**, which may be divided into two separate stages, endeavours to build strength through gradually increasing weights and increasing repetitions, higher-intensity exercises, and then transitioning that increased strength into power and speed. Not surprisingly, this latter stage can also overlap into the next stage where there is a need for race-specific strength building.

- **The race-specific stage** includes recovery, high-intensity interval-based exercises depending on the specific race distance, plus backing off from strength training as the triathlete tapers towards their race. Weights and strength training are usually stopped 2 weeks or more before any important race, depending on your triathlon taper.

- **The maintenance stage** essentially maintains the strength acquired in the weights programme, while focusing on triathlon-specific training for the ongoing competitive season. Emphasis is placed on personal muscular weaknesses and imbalances, addressing any injuries that develop from the ongoing race season, and maintaining core strength. Strength workouts during the competitive season are usually short and specific.

CONCLUSION

The over-riding consideration in any strength programme is that lifting weights that are too heavy for you is the quickest way to get injured, much faster than overtraining or increasing your training volume more than the conservatively safe 10 per cent per week. Muscle strains in the gym as a result of too much weight, too many repetitions or bad technique can happen in an instant. Often they are not discovered until the following day, which means you will probably have continued to train with an injury, invariably making it worse.

The bottom line is that weight training, especially for masters athletes, should be under the supervision of someone who has experience of weight training for masters age groups. This can be your triathlon coach or, more likely, both a personal triathlon coach and a strength coach, perhaps at your local gym.

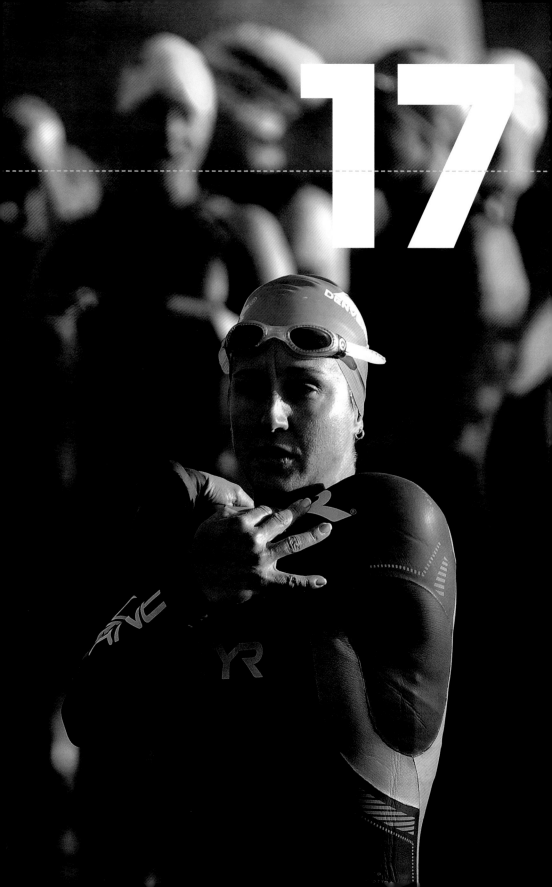

17

PRE-RACE PREPARATION

THREE MASTERS CONSIDERATIONS DISCUSSED IN THIS CHAPTER:

- Preparing to race from the sanctuary of a comfortable environment helps alleviate stress and relaxes the body.
- Get a good night's sleep every day for the entire week leading up to what will probably be a restless last night before the race.
- Reduce the possibility of race day surprises by attending the race briefing and knowing the course in advance.

The final three chapters of this book focus on actual racing: pre-race preparation, race day and recovery. As a result, the advice is not unique to masters athletes, but for any athlete moving up from the beginner level.

Wasn't it Napoleon who said that a good general has the right to be beaten, but never the right to be surprised? We can adapt old Bonaparte's saying and apply it to triathletes: a good triathlete has the right to get their ass kicked by any race course, but never the right to be unprepared.

Pre-race preparation is the place to get all your ducks in a row. It is where you sort out the chinks in your triathlon armour and double-check everything that can go wrong. Because if it can go wrong, there is a good chance it will.

Pre-race preparation is also where you compile checklists; race day is where you implement those checklists. Do not leave it until the night before the race to write out your personal transition area checklists!

This chapter is for non-training pre-race preparation – the things that need to be taken care of in the lead-up to race day. The list can be long and mundane. However, what are covered here are the main topics that should be addressed.

A COMFORTABLE ENVIRONMENT

A triathlete should taper into a race from as comfortable and stress-free an environment as possible. If it is a local race, that should be easy enough. Your home is your castle, so lift up the drawbridge and repel all stress invaders until the race is completed. If you are travelling to a race, creating a stress-free environment can be more problematic. However, turning a hotel room into a stress-free castle is possible as well.

One key is to do everything that needs to be done as early as possible. That way there is no rush to complete required formalities and administration duties later when the lines are longer, the race technology inevitably breaks down and the panic of pre-race chaos sets in. The more that can be completed early, the less there is to stress about closer to race day.

SLEEP

The topic of sleep comes up again! Sleep is the most underrated weapon in a triathlete's armoury, especially for masters, and also the most overlooked. In an ideal world, everyone would get 8 hours of restful sleep the night before a race and be fresh as a daisy on race morning. However, this is not an ideal world and the likelihood is that you will have a fitful night's sleep consisting of just a few hours the day before the race, if that.

Therefore, the best answer to the need for sleep is to make sure you get a good night's sleep, and that means extra hours of sleep as well, every night for the week leading up to the race. If you are fully rested and have had plenty of sleep for the week before the race, a bad night's sleep the night before is something the body can deal with without too much negative fallout. Then, any amount of restful sleep you can then squeeze in the night before the race will be a bonus.

NUTRITION

The subject of nutrition has been covered in detail in Chapter 9 (pages 77–85). As a result, there is no need to repeat the information here. It is sufficient to emphasise that the week before a race is not the time to be calorie counting in an effort to cut that extra half pound of weight. The key to a good race is a healthy diet – allowing for carb-loading – and enough calories to allow the body to function optimally.

REGISTRATION AND CHECK-IN

Registration and check-in is covered more in the next chapter, but the procedures of any race should be taken care of as early as possible to alleviate any unnecessary last-minute stress. To repeat, take care of registration and check-in formalities as early as possible to alleviate any unnecessary last-minute stress. The lines will get longer as you get closer to race day – or race time, if you are registering the morning of the race.

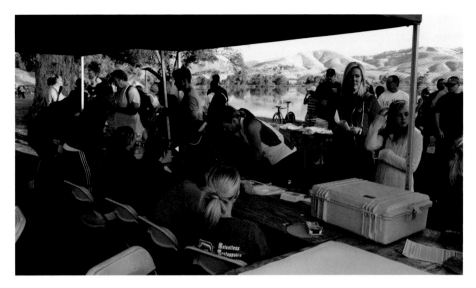

RACE BRIEFING

Even if you are an experienced racer, attending the race briefing is always a good idea. That applies even if you raced the same event last year. Rules change, especially if the race is taking place on public roads or it interacts with the general public or public transport. For example, the local government may have insisted on course changes or procedure changes from last year because of community pressure as a result of traffic congestion. Never assume everything stays the same from one year to the next.

The race briefing is where you will learn about wetsuit eligibility for races with a local water temperature that varies enough so wearing one is contingent on water temperature readings the day before the race. That is something everyone needs to hear first-hand from the organisers, and not second- or third-hand from someone in the hotel lobby!

Along with local rules – which address such things as speed limits downhill – make sure you know the race rules, as they relate to your specific race distance, such as drafting distances or overtaking etiquette. Speed limits can often change from year to year, and can sometimes be implemented the day before a race or the day of a race because of high crosswinds on fast downhill sections.

It is not uncommon for rough seas or sudden ocean swells to change the distance of a swim leg, and even be the reason for cancelling the swim altogether and turning the triathlon into a duathlon.

TRANSITIONS

Even if you pre-register with big races, at most events bike-raking slots are not assigned, although age-group areas will be. That means whoever gets to the transition area earliest on race morning gets the pick of the slots.

You should also take any chance the day before to scout the transition areas for exits to and from the swim and the bike section, the run exit, and distances from the end of each discipline to where you rack your bike. Count the paces and look for any visual markers that you can use to identify where your personal transition area is. At the end of the swim or hard bike, your mind might not be working as well as you would like, and you will be grateful for any visual help in finding your bike in a sea of other bikes that all look the same (i.e. blurred!).

You might be required to set up your bike in the transition area the day before. If so, take all accessories for the transition area with you on the morning of the race and do not leave anything other than the bike overnight. You probably will not be allowed to anyway.

More than likely, though, everything will have to be set up in the transition area the morning of the race. However, you can still walk around and familiarise yourself with the transition area and the location of the starts and finishes of each leg, providing you get there early enough of course.

EQUIPMENT CHECK

Did you check everything on your bike at home before you packed it all into the bike travel case? That is a good start. Check everything again 2 days beforehand, especially on the technical and mechanical sides. Then, to be on the safe side, check everything again the day before. The last thing you need in the countdown to one of your 'A' races are last-minute problems that a more thorough technical check would have detected.

PACKING RACE BAGS

Having gone through your transition area checklists for each of the three disciplines the day before, place everything you need for each discipline on your transition area towel into a separate plastic bag. Then place all the bags into your transition bag, along with warm clothing for when the race ends, and your nutrition needs. Go through your miscellaneous checklist and make sure everything from that is placed into another plastic bag, and pack that into your transition bag as well.

CHECKLISTS

Race checklists are an almost failsafe way of remembering things in the heat of the moment and the intense chaos of a race or pre-race. The swim checklist will be with you before the race. The bike checklist should be taped to the bike somewhere – maybe the frame or saddle – so you can check through it before grabbing your bike and heading for the transition bike exit.

The run checklist can be taped to shoes or something that you know you are not going to forget on the run phase. It is no good taping the list to your fuel

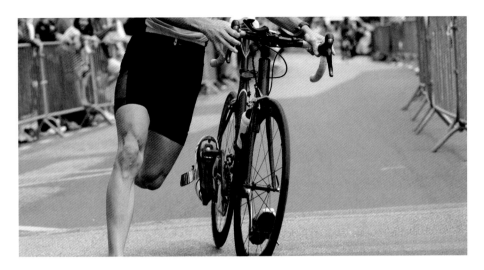

belt if there is a chance you might head off on the run without it. That defeats the purpose of a checklist!

Everyone has their preferences and items that they must include on their race checklists. Some make no sense at all! Others are vital. A triathlete's aging body often has special requirements and preparation that are unique to that person, as well as all the other elements that need to be remembered. As with training schedules, develop your own customised checklists that are unique to your requirements and do not be content with generic, off-the-shelf lists.

What follows, then, are simply suggestions on what an intermediate triathlete should include on the lists for the swim, bike and run. They include only the basics, but personal checklists can, and probably will, get much more detailed and obsessive over the years!

Swim checklist

- Tri suit or swimsuit
- Goggles
- Swim cap (colour-coded, usually provided in race packet at check-in)
- Second swim cap (this one goes on first – then goggles – then race-provided swim cap; two caps keep the goggles securely on your face in the mêlée of the swim)
- Spare goggles
- Anti-fog solution
- Ear plugs
- Wetsuit
- Lubricant to make getting the wetsuit off easier (you will probably be wearing your tri suit under your wetsuit, which will make it easier getting it off your trunk, but not your arms and lower legs)

Bike checklist

- Bike with race pedals attached
- Race wheels or regular wheels (or something in-between?)
- Cycling shorts and shirt (only if you are not wearing a tri suit for the whole race)
- Socks
- Cycling shoes
- Cycling gloves
- Headband or headgear or cycling hat (what are you wearing under your helmet for the cycling section of the race to stop the sweat draining down into your eyes?)
- Helmet
- Sunglasses
- Race number belt (use this for the bike and the run)
- Race number
- Bike computer (to show current speed, average speed and distance ridden)
- Water bottles
- Aero water bottle, with straw and elastic ties
- Spare tube
- CO_2 cartridge and accessories
- Tyre levers and other repair kit accessories that fit in a bag under the bike seat
- Mini pump (are you taking a hand pump as well as CO_2 cartridges?)
- Floor pump (many triathletes take this down to transition check-in for one last tyre pressure check as they place their bike in their slot)

Run checklist

- Running shoes
- Running shorts and shirt (only if you are not wearing a tri suit for the whole race)
- Socks (same as you wore on the bike or different?)
- Fuel belt (longer races will probably require a fuel belt or bottle to go with you – you don't want to leave hydration to chance)
- Hat (what are you going to wear on the run – a baseball-type hat, visor, headband or nothing?)
- Sunglasses (are you using the same ones you wore on the bike?)
- Garmin (or some other wrist-attached electronic device to show your running pace)

Miscellaneous checklist

- Energy bars and gels
- Energy drink
- Salt tablets

- Heart rate monitor (are you using one?)
- Special needs bags
- Sun block
- Toilet paper
- Transition bag
- Towel or mat (for spreading out under your bike in transition)
- Warm clothing (something to change into after the race)
- Pain killers!
- Wristwatch

OTHER PRE-RACE TIPS

Here are some other pre-race tips that might avert a race day disaster!

- Have a pro at a bike shop put on new tubes for your tyres (if you have not changed them in a while), test the brakes and cabling, and generally tune up the bike.
- Put new batteries in all the electronic equipment you are using, such as bike computer, heart rate monitor, Garmin.
- Use a permanent marker to write your name and phone number on all the equipment that at one time or another is going to be lying on your towel in the transition area. Chances are that everything you place on the towel will not stay on the towel and will get kicked and scattered in all directions. Permanent market makes finding all your stuff easier after the race.
- Clip your toenails.
- Know how to get to the start of the race. Do a driving run-through from either your hotel or your home if it is a local race. Time the journey. Figure out where you can park if you are driving to the start. Bear in mind everyone else probably has their eyes on the same parking spot as you!
- Study a map of all three courses: swim, bike and run. See if you can get an elevation map as well so you know where the hills are in advance.

CONCLUSION

Race day can get insane for the unprepared. For the prepared, it should be a relatively calm time, albeit nervous. Pre-race preparation and checklists are the key to lowering stress on race day. Unfortunately, the older you get, the more likely you are to forget some of the myriad details that need to be remembered for the race, and the more you need to develop your own, customised checklists with the things you specifically need. Checklists are therefore all the more essential for the masters athlete.

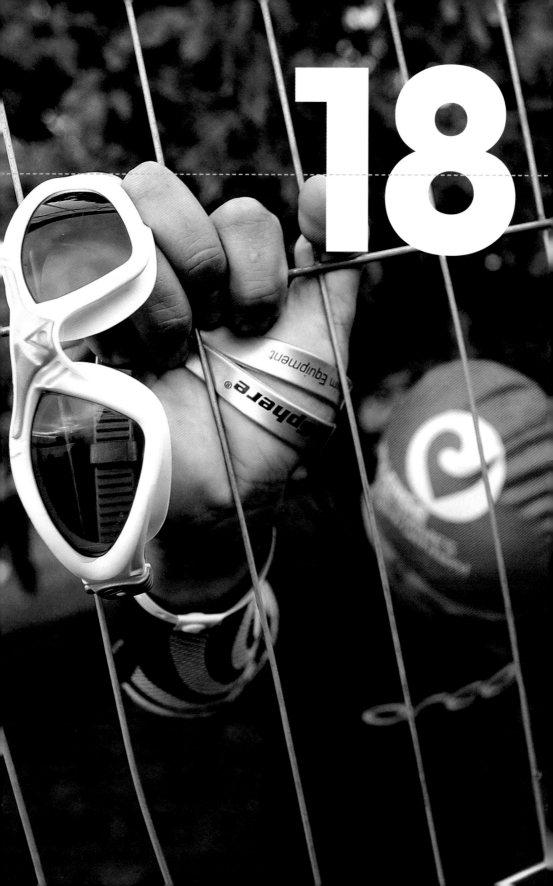

18

RACE DAY

**THREE MASTERS CONSIDERATIONS
DISCUSSED IN THIS CHAPTER:**

- Stress saps energy, which you will need later in the race. So set the alarm clock early to give yourself plenty of time to get ready.

- Whether you are 17 or 70 years old, checklists will save the day, every day!

- For masters especially, even though adrenaline is saying you are ready to go, be sure to warm up properly. If you can't warm up in the water with a short swim, make sure to warm up the upper body, shoulders and arms on land first.

It's go time! Race day is here. The start time is the usual awful crack of dawn. As a result, you have to get up a couple of hours before dawn in darkness. Not that it matters, as you couldn't get any sleep anyway. Now all you want to do is make it to the start line and get on with it.

Not so fast! There are many things that need to be done first. So making a checklist a few days before is a good idea. Once you get into the transition area things will start to get a bit chaotic.

Race day can essentially be broken down into six main areas of focus:

- Getting up and getting there
- Checking in and special needs bags
- Setting up the transition area
- The start
- Nutrition
- Race transitions

GETTING UP AND GETTING THERE
Stay calm and maintain a positive attitude
The main rule on race day is to always stay calm and adopt a positive, 'can do' attitude. You are going to need both from the second you wake up to

the second you step across the finish line, which you will. You can have an emotional breakdown once you have finished!

Start time
The first thing you need to know, and have confirmed directly from the race administration, is your personal start time. If it is a wave start, what wave are you in and what time does it go? If everyone goes at the same time, is it a beach start or is it a water start? Your entire morning revolves around that start time, so be 100 per cent sure you know what it is and where it is.

Set the alarm clock early
Make sure you set the alarm for an early time. Set it earlier than you think you will need. If there is one general rule you need to live by in triathlon, and one that you need to get your head around mentally, it is: 'If something can go wrong, it probably will. So be prepared, physically and mentally.' However, if you do not have enough time to deal with the problem, it doesn't matter how mentally prepared you are. So set the alarm clock early. The worst-case scenario is that you are ready with plenty of time to spare.

When you set your alarm clock late, if you have a major problem – a bike mechanical issue, for example – you will not have enough time to fix it and your race will be over before it begins. You have spent many months preparing for this day, so do not stumble at the final hurdle.

The reality is that few people are going to sleep well the night before a race, knowing they have to get up so early and with so many things that can go wrong. So setting the alarm clock early is unlikely to be interrupting a good night's sleep anyway.

Set two alarm clocks if you can – maybe a watch and a standing alarm next to the bed. If you do not have two alarm clocks, book a wake-up call from the hotel, or even have someone in another country call you at a given time to make sure you are awake, if you are overseas.

Arrive at the race early
Similarly, arrive at the race site earlier rather than later. For the bigger Ironman races, if you do not have to deposit your bike the day before, there will be over 2,000 competitors arriving at T1 to set up their areas and get ready for the start. It will be chaotic. Leave yourself plenty of time to get everything in order and deal with any problems at the race site. Also, if there are no pre-assigned transition spots for age-groupers, the earlier you get there, the better the transition spot you will be able to get (i.e. closer to the end of the row).

What to wear
Most triathlons start at dawn, or soon after. This is to get as many of the competitors around the course, or at least the first part of the course, before

the daily traffic starts to pick up. The less the local public roads have to be closed throughout the day the better. The result is that, even in warm climates, race day starts off chilly, and sometimes downright cold.

So you have to dress appropriately until you strip off down to your tri suit and put on your wetsuit just before the start of the race. Dress in layers, with your tri suit as your bottom layer. In a time pinch, all you have to do is take off the layers and you are already dressed to start the race. As a result, the layers may be tri suit, T-shirt, sweatshirt, sweatpants, warm jacket, warm hat.

Even if you can dress at the race site, remember that so can everyone else. There will be hundreds of people dressing, if not thousands. The one thing you do not want to do is forget your tri suit or swim suit. If you do not have what you need to swim in, again your race is over before it has even begun. Carrying your tri suit to the race site adds another potential problem to an already stressful early morning; it is another bag to carry and another thing to remember. Until you become super-organised and experienced in pre-race nerves, wear whatever it is you are racing in under your other clothes on the way to the site.

Eat breakfast
On race morning, even though you have been carb-loading, you have to eat a breakfast, probably 2 hours before the race start time. It should consist of foods that you are familiar with, that you eat, or have eaten, on regular training days, and for which you have experienced no stomach problems as a result. Even if you have difficulty eating before a race, eat something solid because you will mostly be consuming just fluids and gels for the rest of the day until your race ends. Do not forget that you will be eating nothing for the entire length of the swim. Your first chance will be after the swim, in T1.

Drink
Unlike the other two disciplines, with swimming there is no chance of rehydrating during the race. You have to wait for T1 for that, as you transition to the bike. So make sure you drink adequately on race morning and try to consume a full bottle the hour before the race. On longer races, if you get behind on your hydration at the swim stage of the race you will be playing catch-up all day, and that is not the scenario you want heading into the run.

CHECKING IN AND SPECIAL NEEDS BAGS
Registration
If this is an 'A' race for your season then it is best to take care of registration and/or packet-pick-up as early as possible (i.e. days before). Take care of registration online as soon as you know you are competing in the race. Pick up your packet, containing number, timing chip and so on, at the latest the day

before, to alleviate any stress associated with it. You may have to sign up for a triathlon membership for the day, depending on where you race.

If it is not an 'A' race for your season, and therefore essentially just a training race, you may be able to leave registration until the morning of the race. That said, triathlon races are not like running races where you can just turn up an hour before the start, register and run. Triathlons require a lot of pre-race preparation, such as transition set-up and athlete numbering, so even if it is not an 'A' race for you, take care of as much as you can before race day.

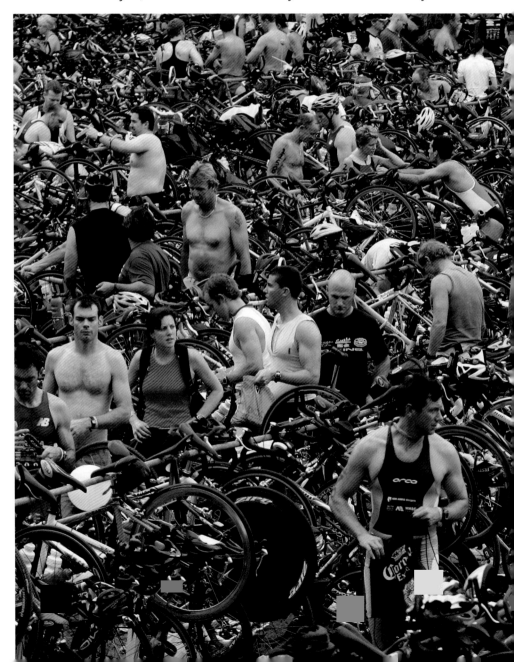

Check-in

Most of the time, if you have pre-registered and picked up your race packet the day before, there really is no race check-in per se. Turn up, set up your transition area, set up your bike, make sure your timing chip has been through the necessary control and race. If, on the other hand, you are registering on the morning of the race, make sure you have taken care of all registration and check-in procedure that is required because you will not have much time.

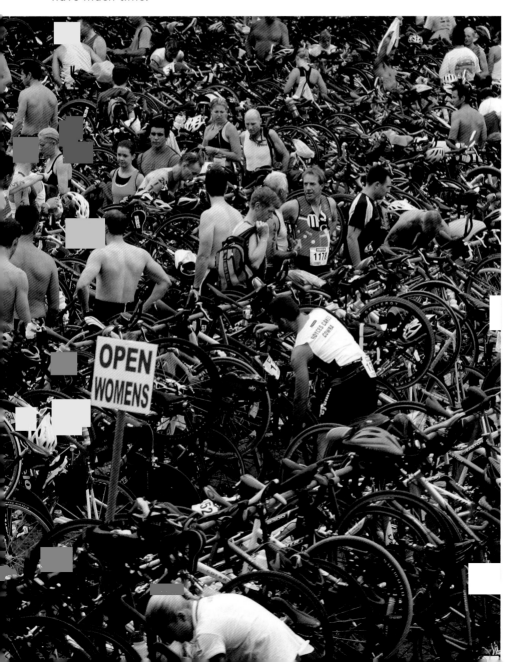

Get numbered on arms and legs

Getting inked with your race number is a time-honoured tradition for all athletes, pros and age-groupers. Take your race number with you and get marked by a friendly person with a stamp or a pen. They may require a photo ID and your triathlon membership details. For the pros, their number is often dictated by their result the year before. Again, get this done as soon as possible after arriving at the race site because the lines get very long the closer the race start becomes.

Special needs bags and transition bag

There is a reason it is called a 'transition bag'. Pretty much everything you will need in transition can fit into it. Many transition bags have a separate waterproof section at the base for a wetsuit. Also, to stay on top of the organisation needed to race a three-discipline sport, place each discipline's gear and special needs in separate bags, and then place them all in the transition bag.

You may need five bags inside the transition bag: Swim gear bag, bike gear bag, bike special needs bag, run gear bag, run special needs bag. In the gear bags should be all the clothing and gear you need for each discipline. When you get to the transition area, they will be easier to unpack and set up.

For the special needs bags, which will usually be available for you at the halfway points on the bike and run courses, there will be certain drop off times and places where you deposit the bags before the race. Find out this information early. For bigger races, this could well be the day before. You only want items in the special needs bags that you absolutely need on the course and cannot get from the food and aid stations. For example, if your special energy gels are actually available at the food stations, don't include them in the special needs bags.

All the special needs and gear bags should go into your transition bag the night before. Even if you are ultra-careful about double-checking, at least it will make the process easier to check on race morning.

SETTING UP THE TRANSITION AREA

Transition deadline

Every race has a deadline time at which point everyone must vacate the transition area. Make sure you know when this is and have set up your area with plenty of time to spare. Double-check you have your swim gear on or with you before leaving the transition area.

The bike

Place your bike in its appropriate slot as soon as you get to the transition area. This is often the morning of the race, but not always. In bigger races, such as some half-Ironmans, for example, you are required to drop your bike off the day before.

I competed in the now-defunct Ironman 70.3 Cancun (it has become the Ironman 70.3 Cozumel) where each transition area bike slot, even for age-groupers, had every registered competitor's name and number already taped to it, so you knew where to put your bike as soon as you arrived.

The bike section of the race is invariably the longest part. However, physiologically, the transition from swim to bike is easier than the transition from bike to run. That is because swimming involves mainly upper body muscles and movement, such as the arms and shoulders, and not the legs. The theory is to save the legs on the swim as much as possible and just utilise the arms and upper body as much as possible, because after the swim, the arms are done for the day. The bike-to-run transition is legs to legs.

There will have been no time to eat or drink during the swim. You will want to do that as soon as you get to your transition spot in T1. As a result, have a bottle of water in the transition area for cleaning sand off the feet before putting on socks and bike shoes, and for taking some mouthfuls before exiting T1. Even though it may not feel like it, the swim will have begun the dehydration process in your body, so fluids will need to be replaced starting immediately.

No need to waste time eating in T1, though. Instead, tape a few gel packets to the frame of your bicycle, either the handbars or the cross frame, and once into your rhythm on the bike, consume some calories.

Also, tape your swim-to-bike transition checklist to your seat. Take a few seconds to go through it before taking it off and exiting the transition area onto the bike course. You want to have a clean, quick transition from swim to bike, but you definitely do not want to leave anything behind.

If there is room in the transition area, pick one side of your spot for bike transition, and the other side for run transition. Then lay out a uniquely colourful towel on the ground beneath your bike, to help you find your bike amid the hordes.

On the bike transition side of your towel, lay out your bike shoes, socks, helmet, sunglasses, maybe a cycling jersey of some sort depending on the weather or the length of race, and your race belt with your race number already fixed onto it.

On the running transition side of the towel, place your running shoes, maybe a different pair of running-specific socks, and whatever type of hat or visor you will be using.

There may be enough room to place back-up items in a gear bag and stuff it under your bike.

Place the bottle of water at the end of the towel with an energy bar and a gel packet, which you can use for either transition if you need to.

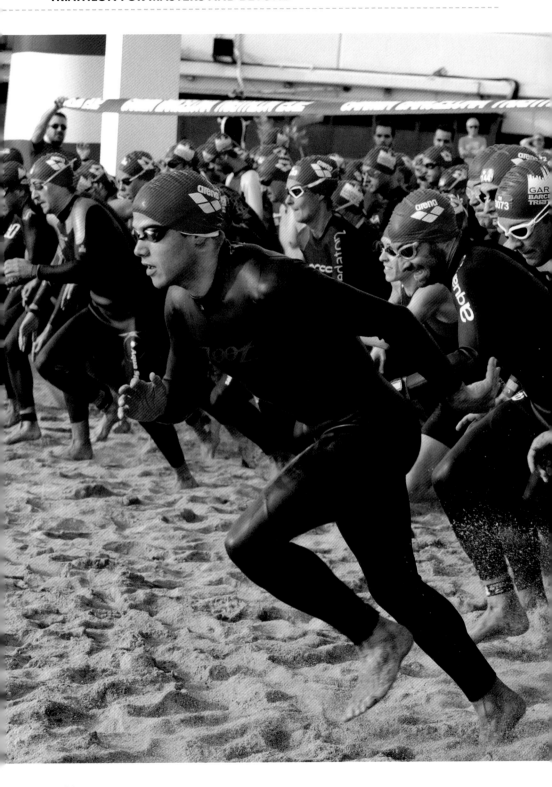

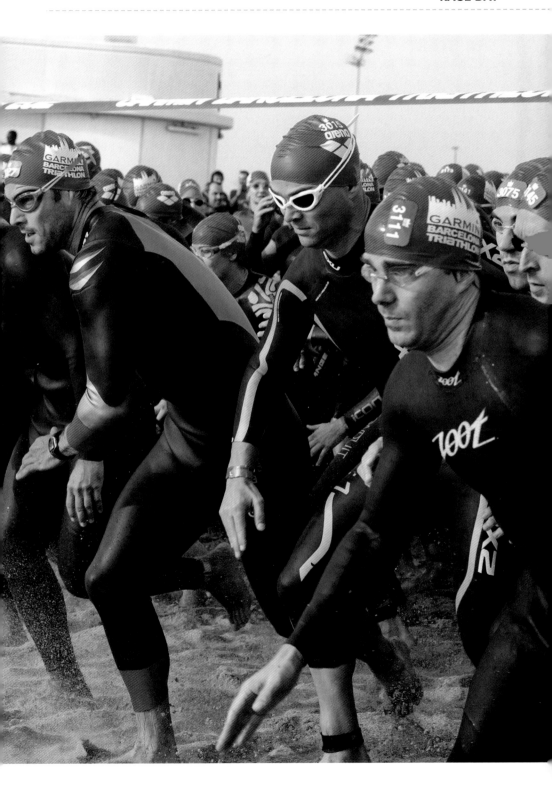

THE START
Warm-up
Leave time for a warm-up. This may or may not be in the water, getting your swim stroke together. However, since the swim is mainly upper-body-focused, it makes sense that the warm-up should involve warming up the arms, shoulders and upper body muscles in some way.

Timing chip
Make sure you know what the organisers want you to do with the timing chip. Do they want you to check in with them at the start line? Do you just have to cross over the chip-timing mat before the start? Do you do nothing at all other than make sure it is attached around your ankle?

Goggles and swim cap
Make sure you have your goggles and swim caps with you in the lead up to the start. Apply anti-fog spray to your goggles while in the transition area. Have your own swim cap on and comfortable before you leave the transition area and head down to the start. Your goggles should be on and adjusted before you enter the water, whether it is a beach start or a swim start. To avoid getting goggles knocked off in the mêlée of the swim, place the age-specific, colour-coded, race-provided swim cap over the straps of the goggles, which in turn are over your own swim cap, so you are wearing two swim caps as a result.

Nutrition
Having eaten a proper breakfast two hours before the start, you should keep hydrated throughout the lead up to the race. Particularly for the longer distance races, you begin the process of dehydration the second the gun goes off and it continues until after you cross the finish line.

Have a sports gel just before you make your way down to the start. Depending on the race distance, you might be in the water a long time. Also, drink a bottle of fluids in the hour leading up to your start, maybe half the bottle with 15 minutes to go. You will get dehydrated in the swim for the longer distances, just as you would on land. There will be no rehydration until you enter T1 in the swim-to-bike transition so make sure you are topped up with fluids to start.

RACE TRANSITIONS
Everyone has their own way of setting up their transition areas – hence the importance of checklists. Go through your checklists and make sure everything is laid out on your towel that needs to be laid out, gels are taped to the bike, checklists are taped to saddles and shoes, and so on.

ALSO ...
Stay positive
To repeat the most important rule of race day: on race day it is essential you stay positive, both before and during the race. Focus on the end-game, which is finishing the race as quickly as you can on the day. Everything else is either there to help you achieve that goal or an obstacle in the way of that goal. There will be physical, mental and probably technical difficulties. You must believe that they can all be overcome.

Stay calm
Coupled with a positive mental attitude is the need to stay calm. If a problem arises, take a deep breath and think of the simplest, most expeditious way to overcome it. An agitated, panicked mind will rush to evaluate and make hasty decisions that could have detrimental consequences a little further down the road. Stay as calm as possible, especially when things are at their most unpredictable.

Rules
Race day is not the time to realise you have not read the rulebook! Better late than never, though. Make sure you are familiar with local race-specific rules, as well as national and organisation rules.

If it is a non-drafting triathlon, make sure you know how many bike lengths you need to be to avoid getting penalised. Needless penalties are always a possibility, but knowing the rules and being able to visually self-implement them under stressful race conditions is essential to a triathlete.

Race your own race
Do not race other competitors. They have their own race plans. You have yours. Stick to your race plan and your own strengths. Be as patient as you need to be to optimise your race performance.

CONCLUSION

There are so many things to remember on race day that it can seem overwhelming. The more you race and practise elements of racing – such as transitions – the less stressful race day becomes. Use whatever organisational aids you can to reduce stress such as checklists.

Be methodical in your execution on race day by staying calm and taking one step at a time. Being prepared limits stress, expedites transitions and consequently improves personal performance.

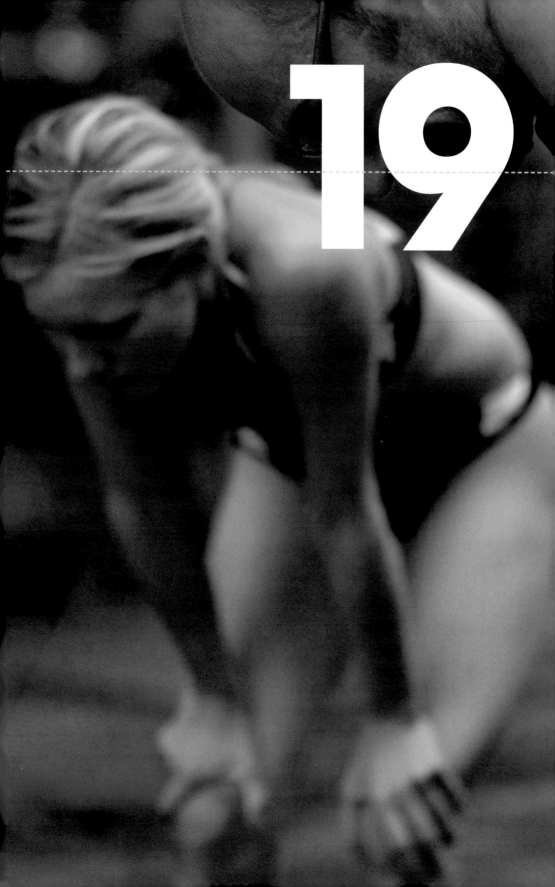

19

RECOVERY

Triathlon is a single sport consisting of three physical disciplines, but five crucial elements for success – swimming, cycling, running, recovery and attitude, with the latter meaning a positive, 'can do' mental approach. It is ironic, then, that recovery, the element that requires the most discipline, is the one that requires the least amount of effort. However, without it, your body will not have a chance to become physically stronger.

In addition, post-race recovery is a dangerous time when your body is at its weakest and most vulnerable to both injury and sickness because of a weakened immune system. As the body ages, the longer it takes to recover, and the more care is needed to ensure a full recovery before training, even light training, begins again. It bears repeating that the body is an engine that needs the right kinds of fuel to function properly, and if you consume foods containing few useful nutrients, then recovery is going to take longer and not be as effective.

Just as in training, a well-executed race recovery programme is essential for any triathlete. This includes muscle recovery and nutrition, along with physical and mental recuperation.

GENERAL RULES OF RECOVERY

Recovery is a very inexact science, whether it is training recovery or race recovery. To make matters worse, what works well for one person can often not work at all for another. That said, there are some fundamentals in the recovery process that can be applied to everyone.

As with all things triathlon and endurance sport, there are dozens (if not hundreds) of books that address the problem to some degree, much of it nutrition-oriented or from an alternative physiological perspective, and some of it so complicated in its language and approach that a PhD in physical education is required just to figure out what it all means!

For the average age-grouper, though, the first rule of recovery is to keep it simple. Or, in keeping with recovery's one-size-does-not-fit-all approach, keep your recovery as simple as you feel you can handle. For some people, the science and research of recovery is enthralling and interesting. For others, it makes their heads explode. The latter just need to know, 'What do I have to do to recover from the race and get back to training?'

For example, estimates as to how many days it takes to recover from a race are just that: estimates. The golden rule of triathlon applies here as well: everyone is different. An often-cited figure is that it requires 3–5 days of recovery for every hour of racing. Therefore, a 2-hour race generally takes between 6 and 10 days to recover from; but it may even be a little more or less.

In addition, as with everything in triathlon, there are some questions to be answered and some details to be filled in before even a realistic ballpark figure can be produced as to a recovery time frame.

So let's go through some of the factors that contribute to recovery times – before, during and after the race.

CONDITIONING AND TRAINING IMPACT ON RECOVERY TIME

Two of the main factors in recovery time are a triathlete's conditioning and what they normally do in training. Obviously, someone who is at their peak of physical fitness training 12 hours a week is going to be able to handle a 2-hour triathlon race better than someone new to the sport or new to structured exercise and who barely trains 6 hours a week.

What type of training you do, coupled with the length of training sessions and their intensity, is also a big factor. If you train in all three disciplines 2 hours or so a day total with varying levels of intensity, a 2-hour triathlon race is not going to seem that much different from a high-intensity daily training session. If a regular training day often involves distances in excess of the race length, then, again, recovering from a 2-hour race should be relatively quick.

That ties in with another factor: race distance. It is usually a lot quicker recovering from a 2-hour triathlon than a 6–7-hour half-Ironman distance. If the 3–5 days recovery per hour of racing figure is applied here, for a 6-hour race it could take between 18 and 30 days to fully recover. The obvious logic is that it will take longer to recover from a longer race than a shorter one.

Another factor is the type of race terrain. A hilly race course is going to have a harsh impact on someone who has primarily trained on the flat. Actually, a hilly course is going to have a considerable negative impact on someone who has also trained on hills! Wind, rain, extreme heat, sun, humidity, crosswinds, rough water for the swim – they are all going to impact recovery time. That applies particularly if you have not trained for those conditions. As a result, race-specific training is paramount.

For the most part, the older the athlete, the longer it takes the average age-grouper to recover. Which means the more careful you need to be with regard to recovery. If a muscle or body part feels tight or sore, even many days after the race and after stretching and massage, hold off another day or so before resuming light training with that muscle group.

A 40-year-old triathlete, and even a 50-year-old triathlete, can still be supremely fit and able to run rings around athletes half their age. However, once 'the big five-oh' has been reached, the downturn in physiology in the average body happens much quicker.

That said, look at the finish time of the 50–54 age group at Ironman World Championship in Kona. The finish times for the top men are unbelievable! But they are not the norm. They are the pinnacle of older age-grouper dreams. That does not mean to say they are not attainable. However, I would venture that there has to have been some serious base endurance work over many years to get to that level.

One statistic from Kona that is more encouraging to older age-groupers is that, in the same 50–54 age group, even a fantastic sub-12-hour Ironman time would not get you in the top 50 triathletes in that age group! That is a lot of athletes maintaining tremendous fitness into their fifties and beyond.

Tying in to the previous comment, experience is going to play a role in recovery, as it does with most things. Someone who has raced dozens of 2-hour triathlons is going to have an easier time recovering than someone who is moving up to the distance for the first time. Whether it is simply the triathlete's knowledge of factors that aid recovery, or that their body is somehow adapting to the high intensities and demands at the distance, is open for discussion though.

That brings us to one of the fundamentals of triathlon: balanced nutrition. Attention to nutrition is almost a product of its time, and in a good way. Thirty years ago, there was barely a book about nutrition and diet for athletes – now there are hundreds. Suffice it to say that the body needs the required fuel, at the right time, to obtain anything like its optimum performance. It is necessary to pay serious attention to nutrition if you want to expedite recovery.

OTHER FACTORS AFFECTING RECOVERY TIME

Other general factors that aid recovery are sleep, compression clothing and fresh running shoes.

Sleep
Sleep is one of the main factors in the aid to recovery, especially for the masters athlete. Getting as much post-race sleep as possible will only help speed recovery. Sleep is the time when the body regenerates and rebuilds most effectively, and if you do not get enough post-race sleep, you are not giving your body the necessary time to rebuild. The result is that recovery can take longer, just by not getting enough sleep. To repeat, the older the athlete, the more important sleep is to recovery.

Running shoes
Fresh running shoes are essential to avoiding injury and speeding up recovery. A new pair, optimally cushioned for you and with the necessary support for your feet, is going to help in post-race recovery. However, new shoes should be purchased a few weeks before a race, so they can be 'broken in'. Never run a race in a new pair of shoes that have not been used over the same race distance in training.

Compression clothing
Compression clothing is not so much a controversial subject as one where elements of its effectiveness are open to discussion. There is extensive research that demonstrates compression clothing such as socks and tights helps in recovery by facilitating blood flow to damaged muscles.

However, many professionals and serious triathletes also use compression clothing, especially socks, during races and training as well. The argument in favour is that, if you know it helps in recovery, why not use it during the race as well in case it helps limit ongoing muscle damage, while also pre-emptively facilitating recovery? What is there to lose?

FREE RADICALS AND MUSCLE SORENESS
Free radicals which are the result of aerobic metabolism – where energy is released from the combustion in cells of oxygen and fuel such as stored carbohydrates (glycogen) and fats – can be damaging to muscles. Antioxidants work to neutralise free radicals and are found both naturally in cells and additionally in supplements. When the natural antioxidants get overwhelmed by the presence of free radicals, supplements are at their most useful.

However, free radicals are also used in a positive way in training adaptation by the muscles to progress to the next level of strength, as well as being less sore the next time they experience the same muscle demands.

The problem is that with too many supplements the body will no longer do its job of producing the antioxidants normally, because the natural signals telling the body to produce them will seem confused. As a result, you should rely more on antioxidants in your diet than on supplements as a way to combat muscle soreness in recovery.

POST-RACE RECOVERY – IMMEDIATE

Practical post-race recovery can be divided up into two main time periods: immediately following the race and then the days and weeks after the race. In this section we concentration on the most important aspects immediately after the race.

Carbohydrate window

There are two most favourable time windows for muscle replenishment after the end of the race:

- within 30 minutes;
- within 2 hours.

Stored carbohydrate in the muscles is called glycogen. If carbohydrates can arrive at the muscles within the 30-minute window, then replenishment is thought to be two to three times faster than if it happens later. The hormone insulin is thought to be responsible for carrying the carbohydrates to the muscle.

A general ratio often used for calorie consumption post-race is two to one in terms of calories to lean bodyweight in pounds. For example, a 100-pound person would consume 200 calories, while a 200-pound person would consume 400 calories.

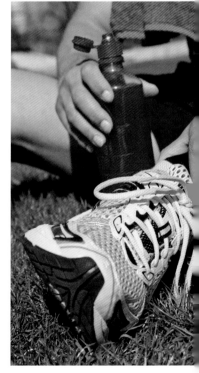

Eating and drinking with a carbohydrate : protein ratio of 4 : 1 has a positive effect on insulin, which, as mentioned, transports the carbohydrates to the insulin-sensitive muscles. Replenishment using the 4 : 1 ratio in the 30-minute window is thought to reduce muscle damage by as much as a third.

Many believe the 'carbohydrate window' extends to 2 hours, although the result will not be as effective as within 30 minutes. At the very least, if you cannot consume your carbs and protein within 30 minutes, aim for the 2-hour mark.

Foods (and therefore carbohydrates) which have a high glycaemic level on the glycaemic index are preferable for recovery, especially in that first 30 minutes. They cause insulin levels to increase quickly in the bloodstream, which aids faster delivery.

Hydration

The longer the course, the more dehydrated you will be. At many long-course triathlon races, such as half-Ironman distances and up, there are medical facilities on site where you can go after the race ends and receive an IV to help rehydrate while you lie down and rest.

Continue to hydrate after the race and into the next day.

Stretching

Do some easy stretching of the hamstrings and quads, and anywhere else that feels tight, as soon as you are able. That means within a few minutes of the end of the race, not just later on in the day. Just as it does at the end of a training session, stretching helps to prevent your muscles tightening up.

Ice

Applying ice to sore muscles immediately after you finish will help. If there is an ice bath in the medical tent, that is also an option as it will both aid muscle soreness and bring your core body temperature down on a hot day. In fact, there is considerable research that says five minutes in an ice bath speeds up muscle healing and cuts down on muscle injury. The longer the race, the more beneficial ice baths become. You won't enjoy the first 3 minutes or so, though! But just remember that your body will love you for it tomorrow!

Protein

Protein is essential to muscle rebuilding. Consuming a big portion of your favourite protein the evening after your race, such as steak or fish, is something to be encouraged, providing your digestion can stomach it of course.

POST-RACE RECOVERY – DAYS/WEEKS AFTERWARDS

There are many factors that contribute to how long recovery takes. The golden caveat is that everyone is different. The ballpark rule, as mentioned earlier, is 3–5 days of recovery for every hour you race. However, there are many pertinent factors.

After that first 24-hour window, the best thing you can do is to control as many of the variables as you can yourself. First come nutrition and hydration. Eat foods that will help you recover – proteins and antioxidants – and drink fluids that will rehydrate your body.

Sleep as much as you can, especially if you are a masters athlete, and try to add an extra hour of sleep every night for a week or so.

Keep moving with some swimming and walking or light cycling. However, do not be tempted to get back into training, even light training, until your body tells you it is fully capable of it.

'Listen to your body' is one of the most used coaching mantras of triathlon. It is used so much because it works. However, it is not just for training. It applies to recovery as well. Go back to training too early and you risk injury, which could delay your real return for weeks.

One word of caution about getting sick, post-race. It is widely known that having a hard race will result in your immune system being depleted for a few days. As a result, you are more likely to catch something like a cold, or another type of bug.

Related to that, there is a family of hormones in your body called interleukins, which direct the body's white blood cells to any area that needs them in order to combat infections and sickness. There have been studies that contend that, following endurance races, such as triathlons and marathons, these hormones are either depleted or disappear almost completely for 36–72 hours, leaving the white blood cells without a road map to any possible infections that crop up. The longer the race, the more the interleukin levels are depleted.

So take special care the few days following a long race to wash your hands continually when out and about, avoiding coughing and sneezing people who are obviously unwell, and perhaps avoiding crowds of people in small spaces with bad air circulation.

CONCLUSION

Recovery is a vital part of triathlon, especially for masters athletes. It is perfectly normal to feel drained of energy and listless, and subsequently unmotivated, for weeks after a race. Time is needed to bring the body back to operating normally again. Lots of rest and good nutrition will help expedite the process. Do not start full training again until your body tells you it is ready. Providing you are eating, sleeping and resting well, recovery will eventually result in a return to form.

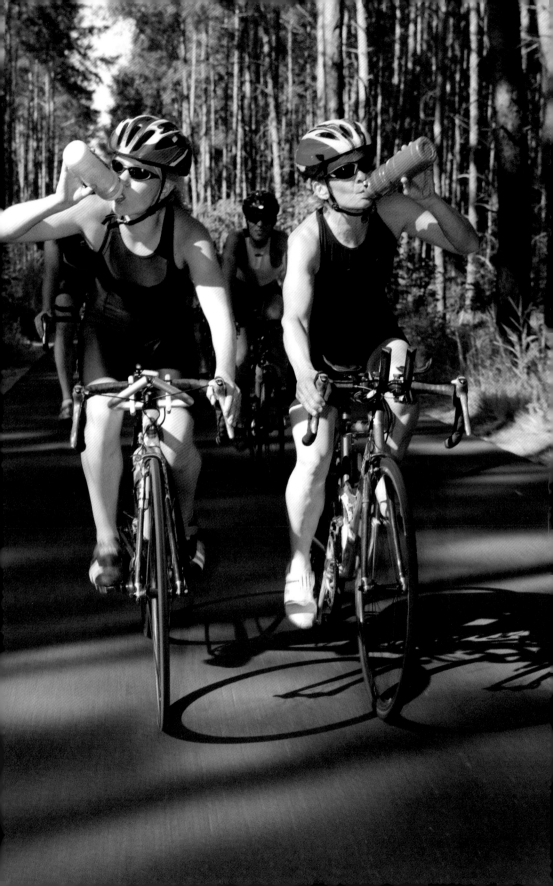

INDEX